THE
NATURAL
— WAY TO —
SOUND
SLEEP

By the same author
The Natural Way to Stop Snoring

THE
NATURAL
— WAY TO —
SOUND
SLEEP

Dr Elizabeth Scott

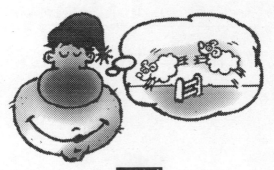

ORION

First published in Great Britain in 1996 by Orion
a division of Orion Books Ltd,
Orion House, 5 Upper St Martin's Lane, London WC2H 9EA

A CIP catalogue record for this book is available from the
British Library.

ISBN: 0 75280 652 1

Typeset at Deltatype Ltd, Birkenhead, Merseyside
Printed and bound in Great Britain by
Clays Ltd, St Ives plc

Contents

Chapter One

What happens
when you go to sleep

You may demand sleep as a right but, like an erection or an orgasm, sleep cannot be forced and may elude your every effort. But is your expectation of how much sleep you need realistic? Many adults retire to bed at 10 p.m. and expect oblivion until eight or nine in the morning. This may be socially and economically attractive. It is not going to happen. Babies, children and adolescents at a growth spurt stage may need up to twelve hours' sleep but once you reach adulthood, seven to eight hours is usually enough.

How do you know if you have had enough sleep?

Are you sleepy by day? If you are, your sleep is not adequate. It may seem long enough, but then its quality must be poor. However long or short your sleep, if you are tired by day you have a sleep problem.

Does this matter?

Not if the sleep lack only lasts a night or two. Everyone has bad nights. You can make sleep up.

Long-term sleep deprivation does matter. You may not notice immediate symptoms, but gradually you become less easy going, readier to fly off the handle; you carry resentments longer and feel down and depressed. When the boss asks for that little bit extra you feel, 'Oh no. I can't do it.'

Chronic sleep deprivation often has a part in causing divorce, child battering and loss of your job.

Many chronically miserable people are simply not getting the right amount, or the right quality, of sleep. Experiments on puppies show that once they have been deprived of sleep for a certain length of time they are unable to make good the loss. Their condition deteriorates and they die.

'So that is just a laboratory test,' you say. 'We don't face this sort of sleep deprivation.'

True, but in this car-borne generation, how many of you have felt sleepy at the wheel?

At a recent meeting of doctors I attended, two-thirds admitted to being dangerously sleepy while driving on at least one occasion. It only takes nodding off for a moment on a motorway to create mayhem. A man did it in front of me the other day. I saw his head go down and his car slewed in front of mine. I braked and hooted. He woke with a start, pulled back into his lane and waved acknowledgement. The crisis was averted. But over a third of motor vehicle accidents are caused by a sleepy driver and of these a significant percentage involve the death of the driver or those he or she hits. It is not enough to be alcohol free at the wheel; you should be well slept and wide awake. Anything less courts disaster.

How do you know you have slept enough?

If you wake well and cheerful every morning, eager to work, happy with your family and friends, raring to go, you are getting enough sleep. This amount might not suit everyone but it is right for you and you should be aware of how much it is, stick to it and insist on it. If you need to catnap during the day, drowse at the wheel of a car or drop off for forty winks if not actively employed, you should do something about your night-time sleep.

What can you do? Keep a sleep diary as a beginning.

Do you have trouble getting to sleep?

Most people fall asleep within half an hour of putting off the light and settling. This is not to say that if you don't, it is abnormal. Some people take an hour to get to sleep yet wake fresh and active for the whole day. This is normal for them. If you are anxious or worried about anything, however, sleep may be long in coming. Your mind goes over and over the cause of your anxiety, round and round like a rat in a trap. Sleep becomes impossible.

Do you have trouble staying asleep?

Many depressed people do. They wake early and cannot get back to sleep. Instead of demanding a sleeping pill from the doctor, discuss the problem. An antidepressant might be more effective. Equally, many old ladies in my medical practice tell me that they go to bed at 10 p.m. and get up at five in the morning. If they are wakeful and active all day, this is perfectly acceptable.

If you wake and sleep, wake and sleep all night, this is unlikely to be normal. It means you are not getting enough of the restorative stages of sleep that your body requires. Many mothers with young children, menopausal women woken by flushes, or snorers and their partners, fall into this category.

Most people with sleep problems have difficulty getting back to sleep if they wake in the night.

Get the answers to these questions straight. Check exactly how many hours you sleep. Assess whether you feel good on waking and if you think you have slept long enough. Be able to tell the doctor how long the problem has

lasted, if you have had it before, and whether
people complain that you snore.

The answers to these questions will allow
your doctor to check that your sleeplessness is
not due to any accompanying illness. Then you
can confidently search for a cure from the many
offered by this book, both from a Western
medical approach and from the treatments
offered by practitioners from other countries
and other disciplines.

The idea that sleep was a sort of descent into
oblivion changed in 1928 when Hans Berger, a
German psychiatrist, recorded changing electrical activity on electrodes attached to the scalps
of sleeping people. The electroencephalograph
was born. Since then, knowledge of what is
going on in your brain and body while you sleep
has moved on rapidly. Sleep stages have been
defined according to the sort of brain wave
recorded by the electroencephalograph and doctors are aware of what is a normal, healthy
tracing and what is not.

When you shut your eyes and drift into sleep
you pass first into stage 1 of non-rapid eye
movement sleep (non-REM sleep), so called
because your eyes lie inert behind your lids. This
sleep deepens. On an electroencephalograph
tracing taken from electrodes attached to the
face and head you can see that the irregular, low
waves of stage 1 begin to show sudden peaks

and spindle-shaped wave patterns. These are characteristic of stage 2 non-REM sleep. As this deepens, the brainwaves slow and become larger. Stage 3 is where these large, slow waves occupy 20 per cent of the trace and stage 4 is where they occupy 50 per cent of the trace.

In stage 4 you are fast asleep. You can be roused but with great difficulty and you feel almost disoriented when you come to. Remember the feeling of being woken about twenty minutes after you have fallen asleep? You felt positively unwell. You were probably in stage 4 non-REM sleep.

From stage 2 it is easier for you to be roused, especially if your name is called, and stage 1 sleep is that pleasant stage of drowsiness reached in a boring lecture or concert or when you nod off in front of the television. Reality just slips away and you lose chunks of the action around you. Sounds are maximized; a tinkle of a teaspoon wakes you as if a drum was being played.

Stages 1 and 2 non-REM sleep seem just to be time-fillers. They may, however, have some function in diffusing stress and later on in this book I will describe how they are summoned to perform this function. Stages 3 and 4 non-REM sleep (deep sleep stages) are the times when growth hormone is released into the body to help the young grow and the older person repair tissue damage. 'You'll feel better after a good sleep' is not just an old wives' tale.

Melatonin, another hormone secreted by the pineal gland, has been found to assist in getting you to sleep. I shall be discussing this naturally occurring hypnotic later.

As night goes on, the hormones prolactin and cortisol are also secreted into the bloodstream to be carried round the body. These form a sort of wake-up jag that allows you to wake, raring to go. For these hormones alone a good deep sleep is essential.

Usually you slip quite quickly into the deeper stages of sleep. Then, after about an hour and a half, your sleep lightens for a while and may go into the stage of rapid eye movement sleep. The electroencephalograph trace from the scalp shows a small irregular wave pattern and the leads over the eyebrows show that the muscles around your eyes are very active. All the rest of your muscles lie flaccid, almost paralysed, except for the diaphragm, that great bellows of a muscle that separates your chest from your abdomen. It does your breathing for you during REM sleep while the muscles around your ribs do not move. You can see the eyes of a person in REM sleep squinting and rolling. Babies under three months old drift in and out of REM sleep and their eye movements behind their lids are very obvious; not surprising when you realize that REM sleep seems to be the time when the brain is looking after itself. A baby's nervous system is comparatively undeveloped at birth though the body is completely formed. It seems reasonable that REM sleep plays a large part in a baby's development.

In adult life it is in this part of sleep you are most likely to dream. Your brain is sorting itself out for the next day. Unwanted information is being lost, feelings and learning acquired through the previous day are being given their proper importance. The circulation to your brain in REM sleep is greatly increased.

So in a normal night you fall asleep within half an hour, pass rapidly into deep sleep, stay there for an hour and a half before you reach a lighter stage, and then either return to deep sleep or move into REM sleep for another period of an hour and a half with the stages following each other and gradually lightening until you wake in the morning.

The time in each stage is governed by your inbuilt daily clock, your ultradian rhythm, whose motivator lies deep in the mid-brain. All through the 24-hour day you get restless and need a change of pace every 90 to 120 minutes. Through the day you may get up from your desk, stretch, have a cup of coffee, then get back to work, stop for lunch, have a cup of tea and be ready to go home for supper. This broken regimen continues through the night as you change sleep stages. Until doctors saw encephalograph tracings through sleep they had no idea of this continuing cycle. They knew about the sleep–wake cycle, the circadian rhythm that operates to make you sleep at night and wake by day. It controls your temperature and sleepiness so that at night your temperature drops as you go to sleep and rises as you wake.

You also have a secondary period of temperature drop and sleepiness around midday till two in the afternoon. The siesta is not just a habit; it is encouraged by the controls in your brain. The western world tends to ignore it but it can be very useful to adjust disordered sleep patterns or to make up lost sleep or to diffuse stress.

Doctors now search for the chemical reactions that trigger the cells that cause sleep and its various stages. Serotonin, norepinephrine and acetylcholine have all been found to be neurotransmitters, controlling the brain cells' ability to fire electrical impulses and so induce sleep or wakening. How and where they work is still not completely known but this will not be long delayed and then perhaps a sound night's sleep will be easily available.

Until then what interests the sleepless is not why they are sleepless but how they can get a decent night's rest.

I have brought together treatments from

many countries and from other therapeutic traditions as well as my own to allow those who cannot sleep to find some treatment that might work for them. Hypnotic medication may be frowned upon but it has a place, especially in the short term, and I have explained the currently available medicines and how they work so that you may be able to assess which, if any, will suit you.

First you need a checklist of dos and don'ts to make sure that some simple step to getting a good sleep is not being forgotten. There are many such lists available, called 'Sleep Hygiene' leaflets, a bad name as these are little to do with washing yourself but more to do with cleaning up your pre-sleep act. This is my one:

1. Assess how much sleep you need to remain active and wakeful through the day and see that you get it. You may have to experiment with going to bed half an hour earlier or later, or getting up half an hour later or earlier until you have it right. You cannot move your sleep time by more than half an hour without finding difficulty so do this gradually. This may be time-consuming but is essential. The amount of sleep you needed as a child is often very different from what you need in old age and awareness of this will stop you thrashing

around in bed expecting nine hours' sleep or more when you have already had quite enough.

An honest assessment of how much time you really sleep is also vital. Many people have asked me for sleeping pills because they have not had a wink of sleep when in fact sleep studies show that they slept well most nights. This feeling comes from drowsing in and out of the lighter stages of sleep, often because of anxious thoughts which follow you into sleep and are present on wakening. Your sleep is not so much absent as of the wrong kind to provide real rest. The chapter on stress will offer help with these problems.

People whose hours vary from day to day, such as travellers through time zones or shift workers whose shifts change daily, have a separate problem. In the case of the jet-lagged and for those subject to short-term shift changes, the best answer is to 'crash out' for two hours on arrival or on finishing work. Use an alarm clock to wake up after this and then accept the current time zone for the local area.

Shift workers whose shifts run for longer periods will find transition easier if the shifts move forward round the clock, and this is worth negotiating with the boss. Disturbed nights do follow a shift change so it is much better to have a considerable period in each shift rather than quick changes. Use the normal circadian tendency to sleep from 10 p.m. to 3 a.m. at night and midday to 2 p.m. in the afternoon to assist the change and through this book you may find helpful techniques that work for you. Meditation to slow down, homeopathic remedies, acupressure and herbal therapy may all help and in the end a sleeping pill that does not alter your sleep pattern for the first night of the change will not cause addiction: one of these, say every three months, might just allow a good day's work on shift change.

2. Go to bed at the same time each night and also get up at a set hour. Use an alarm clock to wake to if necessary. If you have got to know how many hours' sleep you need, then that should be your regular stint.

A patient of mine came in complaining that she was exhausted in her new job. Was the promotion too stressful? No. She craved the extra responsibility. She was tired. What about sleep times? She went to bed regularly at 11 p.m. and she knew she needed eight hours. So had anything changed in the morning? Yes, she now had to catch a 7 a.m. train to work so got up earlier. Where were the eight hours? She changed her bedtime, went to bed an hour earlier through the week, kept her weekends for going out at night and late sleeping and in a month was full of energy. She had suffered the effects of chronic sleep deprivation. The body learns to fall asleep at the same time each night if we get a regular time going.

3. Avoid eating or drinking stimulating substances for at least four hours before bedtime. Everyone knows that coffee and tea keep you awake, so avoid them at night. Decaffeinated tea and coffee often contain some residual stimulating substances and these drinks encourage urination, so even they may not be advisable late at night. A hot milk drink or barley water is often a help in getting to sleep. Many fizzy soft drinks do have caffeine in them, and so should be avoided.

What about alcohol?

A single drink may relax you and make you sleepy. It probably does not have much more effect. However, more than one drink may disrupt your sleep pattern and wake you early, often in some discomfort with headache and nausea. It may also become addictive so should not become a regular part of your pre-sleep habits.

Herbal teas will be discussed later in more detail as they are becoming readily available in the shops. Some of these, like dandelion and ruibos, are diuretic so are not suitable at night; others like camomile or hibiscus may be soporific but produce wild dreams for some people, so should be treated with caution as a late-night drink.

It is worth minimizing any late-night fluid intake if you do not want to get up often to pass urine.

Heavy, fat-laden meals are not conducive to a good night's rest. 'Breakfast like a prince, lunch like a lord and dine like a down-and-out' is good advice. I wish all hostesses would take note. Fats take a couple of hours to be digested in the stomach and your system is still busy trying to cope with the cream and butter of a gourmet dinner as you are trying to get to sleep.

Regular medication should also be checked to make sure it is suitable to be taken at night. For instance, diuretics, which encourage urination, should be taken in the morning. Some antidepressants are stimulating and should not be taken at night. Vitamins should be taken with breakfast so they can act through the day. In fact, if your sleep becomes less good after starting a night-time medication, it is worth switching it to the morning if possible to see if a normal sleep pattern returns.

4. Keep the bedroom for sleep and sex. A bedroom full of the stomach-gurgling smells of a fish supper does not encourage sleep. If you live in a bed-sitter, open the windows to clear the air before bedtime. Watching television may

make you nod, but turn it off and turn over and the brain leaps awake. A book read before switching off the light seems to be more soporific.

Make sure the room is as quiet as possible. In cities the ambient noise is much greater than in the country, but you get used to it. Strangely, subliminal noise is a greater irritant than the sound of buses passing the house. This may be the ticking of a clock, or the rattle of a pipe or the vibration from the fridge of an upstairs neighbour. Once heard it is unforgettable and sleep becomes impossible. It should be tracked down and stopped. Pipes can be lagged, equipment can be given rubber pads underfoot: subliminal noise can and should be stopped.

Your bedroom should be comfortable, neither too hot nor too cold. It should not have computers and work apparatus around to keep your mind from sleep. If they have to be present, they should be put away or covered, offering no temptation to do 'just a little bit more'.

5. Your bed must be comfortable. You spend nearly a third of your life in it, renewing your strength for the day. The mattress, the bed covers, the pillows are all important. They must give you a feeling of relaxation when you get into bed. Everyone has different needs, and these should be met. If you are asthmatic or a

hay fever sufferer who is allergic to feathers, check that the filling of your pillow, duvet and mattress is of artificial fibre; if you twitch or move about while asleep you might sleep better in a single bed. Money spent on a comfortable bed is well spent. There is an old wives' tale that suggests that you sleep better if your bed lies on a North-South axis. I have heard it so often now that I believe it may have relevance for some people. If sleep is hard to come by in a new bedroom, consider it.

6. Make sure your room is dark. Summer and full moon nights can bring poor sleep to those who need a comfortable blackness around them. Light can be as annoying as sound.

7. You will sleep if you are tired enough. Heavy exercise last thing at night stimulates a rush of adrenalin into the bloodstream, which tends to wake you up, but unless you have enough exercise you are unlikely to sleep well. Walking to work and back, lunch-time exercise classes or swimming, early evening brisk walking or cycling or jogging all help to clear the stress of the day from your mind and tire your body.

8. Don't make major decisions late at night. Your brain will not switch off. A good row at bedtime is sleep defeating. In the chapter on

stress and in the chapters on different medical approaches I have listed many techniques to unwind overactive minds, but it is preferable to enter sleep at ease with the world. You need a routine that signals your brain to switch off. Do your teeth, say your prayers, get into bed and read a book or switch off the light and play some music. I am so convinced that music helps that I designed three cassettes of classical music to run at the brainwave rate of people as they fall asleep and this 'Sound Asleep' series for babies, adults and seniors has proved a boon to those who have difficulty just 'getting over'.

9. Catnap if it helps you to avoid sleep deprivation. If it is just a reaction to boredom, avoid it by filling your day with interest or activity or both. However, many of you have such mentally or physically tiring jobs that you need to 'crash out' during the day. The obvious time is the noon to 2 p.m. blip in your circadian rhythm, when you are programmed to sleep for a while. Many hot countries have their work pattern set to accept a siesta in the middle of the day. This seems to me entirely reasonable. Some people boast that they only need four or five hours' sleep, but have taught themselves to drop into deep sleep for half an hour here and there through the day. In this way, they allow their bodies to get the right amount of deep sleep to

stay healthy. So catnap if you need to. It won't affect your sleep unless you are turning day into night through boredom.

10. Go to bed when you feel sleepy. This time may not suit the rest of the house, but if you have trouble with sleep the other inhabitants should be sympathetic and allow you quiet. Many of my patients sit watching their televisions, drowsing on and off until everyone decides it is bedtime. They then go to bed and find they are unable to get to sleep. They have fought their body clock's switch-off time and found themselves beginning to wake up when they put their heads on the pillow. Listen to your body clock.

11. No sleep hygiene routine would be complete without mentioning sex. Having intercourse is one of the best soporifics known to man. A loving relationship fully consummated leaves both parties happy and relaxed. Even masturbation, though it is frowned on by many religions, may bring comfort to some.

12. An older patient said to me the other day, 'My friends all talk about being unable to sleep because of stress but I just say my prayers and shut my eyes and feel content and sleep comes.' I promptly added religion into my sleep hygiene

leaflet. Say your prayers last thing and go to sleep. If you are deeply religious you will probably want to pray at an earlier time, when you can concentrate; but last thing at night, if you have a belief, it is very comforting and stress relieving to offer your whole self and your loved ones to the care of the God you believe in or reinforce the 'peace that passeth all under-standing' that is the goal of most religions. The fear of death that so often visits at night may be assuaged by prayer and those of you who grew up in a faith but forgot it when the world opened before you might consider the comforts of religion, any religion.

If you are not religious, block wakeful thoughts using some of the techniques in this book. Serious or anxious thoughts will prevent sleep taking over your brain. Banish them and sleep will come in the natural way it is meant to.

Summary

And so to bed
Samuel Pepys

1. Go to bed at the same time every night and rise at the same time every morning. Look for the time when you feel sleepy at night and go to

bed then. This reinforces your natural sleep-wake rhythm. Catnaps in the afternoon are fine if you are used to them.

2. Make sure your bed is comfortable, your bedroom dark, quiet, not too hot or cold or damp – a pleasant, welcoming room.

3. Establish a set going to bed routine to prepare your mind for sleep, e.g. have a shower, do your teeth, set the alarm clock for the morning, get into bed, read a book, put out the light, switch on your tape recorder and follow the sound of your 'Sound Asleep' cassette into sleep.

4. Keep the bedroom for sleep (and sex). Cover work surfaces and computers at night. Don't leave food remnants about.

5. Avoid wakening substances such as coffee, tea, nicotine and rich foods late at night. Remember, alcohol may make you sleepy but wakes you early. Barley water or a warm milk drink may help you get to sleep.

6. Exercise earlier in the day. At night, gentle exercise and relaxation exercises are appropriate.

7. Block wakeful thoughts using a technique from this book.

Chapter Two

Organic causes
of insomnia

You take sleep for granted until it doesn't come.
It would do so if you were in perfect health, well
fed, well exercised and lying in a comfortable
bed with a quiet mind. Modern living has made
a monkey of these simple requirements. Shift
work, travelling, or jet lag take time to adjust
to. Double beds, while fun, are not always
peaceful to share. You go to work by car or
public transport, stand about or sit in front of a
computer or desk all day. You may get stiff
muscles and tired legs, but the weight on the
eyelids that follows hard physical exercise is
gone with childhood. It is amazing how you still
sleep well unless there is something wrong.

The most important question I can ask my
patients in surgery is 'How are you sleeping?' If
the answer is 'Not well', and especially if the
insomnia is recent, I know I must search

carefully for signs of early disease before I put it all down to stress.

What illnesses affect your sleep? Let me list a few common ones.

Gastric ulcers traditionally wake sufferers with hunger pains in the middle of the night. At first the pain is relieved by antacids or a glass of milk and a biscuit, but if this pattern emerges it is better to get curative treatment from a doctor.

Irritable bowel disease, once diagnosed, receives little further help than dietary advice. Yet it may wake you with a feeling of abdominal discomfort that keeps you awake for hours. Twenty years ago the treatment was to eat only soft food; now doctors prescribe plenty of roughage. Neither do much to soothe the annoying bowel discomfort. In my experience the condition is often due to a food intolerance and the big three causes are intolerance to chocolate, coffee and milk products, with wheat products a hot fourth. A three-month trial minimizing these products, while maintaining a balanced diet, is sometimes an easier way to return to a good night's sleep.

Sometimes we know what food doesn't suit us. It is often one that we are very fond of. I had a patient whose problem was smoked salmon. He had had trouble for twenty years. I could scarcely credit his food intolerance result when I saw it, but he shamefacedly admitted he adored the stuff and ate it most days. Stopping it for six months solved his problem and he returned to eating it occasionally and enjoying it without discomfort. Excluding substances you are intolerant to for a while and then bringing them back into the diet in small quantities works for many people.

Patients with hiatus hernia, where their diaphragm allows abdominal contents to push up into their chest area, should not sleep on high pillows. This just creates more upward pressure. They should raise their bed heads up on 4-inch (15cm) blocks and use one pillow. This way, stomach contents tend to be kept in their proper place by gravity.

You should not disregard abdominal pain that wakes you in the night. Gall stones, appendicitis, intestinal obstruction and tumours may all start this way.

All forms of heart disease cause restless sleep, which is not good news for the sufferer because what he or she really needs is the deep restorative sleep that aids recovery. Sometimes patients with heart failure report Sisyphian dreams of heavy labour, such as pushing a great weight up a hill. They wake breathless and miserable. Most doctors will see to it that their patient's sleep pattern is restored, even if it means giving a short-acting sleeping pill until the crisis is over. A normal sleep is obviously preferable, so all the normal sleep hygiene requirements are doubly important when a person has heart problems. If high pillows help, then they should be comfortably arranged. Relaxation exercises and foot massage, which are discussed later in this book, or a change of clothes and a washdown or bath before bed are all helpful.

High blood pressure often causes increased waking through the night. People wake with their jaws clenched against the pressure and a morning headache is a frequent feature. Getting your blood pressure checked is simple, and it may be life saving.

Angina may sometimes be troublesome at night and heart attack should always be suspected if the pain persists. This sort of pain should be treated as an emergency and a doctor summoned.

Patients with early cancers often sleep less soundly, giving the pattern of early morning wakening or the repeated wakening through the night that depression gives. If a patient of mine becomes depressed for no good reason and especially if he or she begins to lose weight, I may treat the depression but I also look repeatedly for signs of an early cancer.

People with chest trouble have disturbed nights because they are woken by cough. High pillows often help chronic bronchitics, but treatment of the underlying condition is essential.

Smokers who give up often have a period of loose chronic cough for about three months after they stop. This has to be accepted and is self-limiting.

Poorly controlled asthmatics wake coughing through the night and are breathless in the morning. Asthma is a disease where the lung passages constrict and become inflamed. It is thought to be in part an allergic reaction to the house dust mite, but may be exacerbated by stimuli such as stress or animal fur or infection. It is often familial. I am always amazed at how much wheeze asthmatics will put up with. They should not have to do so at night. In all but the mildest asthma you should have medication to subdue both the constricting force and the inflammation in your lung passages. This is an affliction where you should work closely with your doctor and you should choose a doctor who is interested in asthma control. There are good medications available, but you must feel comfortable about taking them or you will tend to 'forget' the dose. Get your doctor to tell you about all the available medicines and ways of taking them and work out with him a combination that suits you. It is worth getting asthma medication right and being aware that if you begin to lose sleep or wake breathless, you need medical reassessment at once.

Asthma is a growing problem. Specialists are not entirely sure why. They suggest that stress, urban pollution or increased use of propellant sprays might have something to do with it. Sometimes where we live may influence the disease. I had a patient who holidayed in Egypt and found his asthma disappeared while he was there. He was so much struck by this finding that year by year he took his holidays there and found the same healing. It may have been loss of stress in his life but he was convinced it was the dry air. Indeed, in Victorian times, if you had a bad chest and were rich enough, doctors recommended wintering in Egypt.

It is not possible for all of you to emigrate to a dry atmosphere, but you can keep your bedrooms free of sprays, scent, powder, and dust. For an asthmatic, a good night presages a good day.

Stress has an effect on asthma. I had an older patient who became asthmatic when her daughter left her house to marry. She did not like living alone and began to wheeze when she felt upset. Eventually she needed a great deal of medication to control her wheeze. When she became very old she became demented. She was no longer stressed and her need for an inhaler ceased.

Itch, for whatever cause, is another sleep destroyer. Patients often feel it is too trivial a

matter to trouble their doctor with and put up
with restless nights, scratching. Most itches
have a cause that can be cured and if not there
are antihistamine creams and medications that
may help as short-term prescriptions. Because
eczema is sometimes hard to control, even with
all the medications available to allopathic doctors, patients and doctors are turning to other
disciplines such as homeopathy, herbalism and
Chinese medicine to see if they have an effective
alternative.

One interesting modern disease is the dry skin
itch that accompanies the installation of central
heating. Keeping your skin well moisturized is
the cure here.

Pain is a great sleep destroyer. Discomfort of
any kind from a frozen shoulder and the
'rheumatics' of old age, to more serious causes,
can keep you awake. Even without curing the
cause, just getting rid of the pain is enough to let
you relax and sleep well. It is worth trying
physiotherapy, acupuncture, massage and other
simple remedies before resorting to painkillers.
However, if a couple of aspirin or a paracetamol will offer a sound sleep and a good day,
especially in older people, I cannot see any
reason not to take them. You have to accept
that there may be side effects. Aspirin may cause
gastric bleeding and paracetamol may damage

the liver, but where you accept that the result is worth the risk, you may want to take it.

Men, as they get older, have frequent wakenings and difficult micturition because of prostate enlargement. Nowadays there are medical as well as surgical treatments, so there is no need to fear a visit to the doctor.

Early diabetes may cause the need to urinate more often both day and night, as well as causing thirst.

Women often sleep less well premenstrually for a day or two and may well need relief for painful periods. Aspirin with its anti-inflammatory effect, or a codeine-based medication which relieves spasm, may be effective in the short term but continuing pain and heavy periods require further investigation and medical treatment.

Menopausal sweats can make nights dreadful. Heat, excitement and alcohol all encourage menopausal sweating so a cool bed, cotton nightwear and a handy change of clothes all help. Hormone replacement therapy is very effective and may also prevent later osteoporosis and brittle bones. However, it has its own side effects, so it becomes a personal decision whether to put up with some months of poor sleep or accept medication.

Gland disorders may show first in sleep disturbance. Thyroid over- or under-action often brings a patient to the doctor complaining that their sleep pattern has changed.

Any infection, especially when accompanied by fever, will make sleep difficult and patchy. You all know the joy of the deep sleep you get as soon as you begin to recover from a viral illness such as influenza.

Depression as an illness usually starts as a change in your sleep pattern. Sometimes you wake early and cannot get back to sleep; more often you wake repeatedly through the night as well. It is worth considering whether your general outlook on life has become more gloomy. Do you feel less able to cope, worthless, unable to go into company? Have your moods become unstable and your eating habits variable?

If you are suspicious that you may be becoming depressed ask a close friend. They often see changes before you can accept them. Depression cures best with early treatment, either through your own efforts or with help and treatment from a doctor. Your sleep pattern will return to normal once the depression is under control.

Any illness has some effect on your sleep and disturbed sleep may be the first sign of malaise, so an unexplained change in sleep pattern that persists for more than two weeks is worth a visit to the doctor. Eye pain from glaucoma, headache from sinusitis or earache from infection:

there are many causes of sleep loss which need a doctor's investigation and treatment. Even the slimmer sleeps less well while his or her weight drops.

However, most people know why they are not sleeping. They just don't know what to do about it. Through this book I shall be describing different ways to help you go to sleep and get a full night's sleep without having to take medication regularly. I hope I shall have offered a lifeline to everyone who reads on, but if you have to take medication, even for a short time, you should know what you are taking and how it affects you.

The sap of the opium poppy has long been known for its soporific effect. Opiate derivatives are strong hypnotics and pain relievers. Morphine and heroin, to name but two, are used in medicine for very ill patients who need these effects. They are not available over the counter and although they have become widely used drugs of addiction, they are not to be classed as simple sleeping pills.

When I entered general practice the strongest medicine we offered patients to help them sleep were barbiturates. Sodium amytal and Soneryl were commonly prescribed. These were habit forming, partly because if stopped after having become accustomed to them, the taker became very disturbed and often hallucinated, very much as an alcoholic does when he or she suddenly stops alcohol. Once recognized, doctors and patients turned to other hypnotics and the benzodiazepines became popular: long-acting nitrazepam and the shorter-acting temazepam. Although the longer-acting antianxiolytics such as diazepam have become less prescribed because they also were found to be addictive, temazepam has become a very commonly prescribed hypnotic. It is effective but as patients get used to it they sometimes need greater doses and the carry-over sedation can then extend into the next day. Its chief problem is that, like all the benzodiazepines, it suppresses rapid eye movement sleep. As this is the time when your brain appears to renew itself, it is a serious side effect. Eventually REM sleep breaks through to some extent, but then if you stop temazepam you get an enormous amount of dream-disturbed sleep as the brain tries to make up for lost time. This usually brings you back to the doctor saying that your sleep is no better and you need more pills. You should know that if you take temazepam or any of the benzodiazepines for even a week, you are likely to have disturbed sleep for a couple of weeks after you stop and must be prepared to put up with this for the short term benefit you needed. Addicts have long abused temazepam, so it has become a listed drug and as such will be prescribed less and less for even short-term insomnia. It joins the opiates as a hypnotic to be used in serious illness.

An alternative has been the use of antihistamines. Some of these are more sedative than others. They tend to be cheap and available without a prescription, but are often long-acting, especially in the elderly. This may mean that if you take them at night you could still feel sleepy next day. They tend to act more slowly than other sleeping pills, so it is essential not to take too much in the hope they will act more quickly. They do not. Overdosage may make you feel restless rather than sleepy and serious overdosage may give you hallucinations.

Chloral in various forms is another sedative that your doctor may suggest. It has been around a long time, so doctors know a lot about its side effects. It causes dependence and, in higher doses, may cause indigestion and delirium. For these reasons I feel that it should, like the benzodiazepines, be treated as yesterday's medication and unless there is a very good reason to prescribe it, I prefer to use one of the newer sleeping pills. Chlormethiazole is a similar old-fashioned hypnotic whose side effects in my opinion outweigh its benefits, and I would only use it where nothing else would do.

Doctors and the general public have got into

a state where they treat insomnia as a disease to be cured. It is not. It is a disturbance of your normal daily pattern of life and, except where incurable illness is present, if you remove the sleep-preventing factor, your own body will bring you sleep at the expected time. Therefore you should see sleeping pills as necessary only in the short term to allow you to rectify a state hostile to sleep and you should make sure that the sleeping pills you take do not have side effects that make more trouble for you than the reason for which you took them.

Two new pills fit this bill. Zopiclone and zolpidem are both short-acting, effective sleeping pills that do not disturb the normal pattern of your sleep. In fact, the zolpidem manufacturers even suggest that their product increases the deep, body-restorative sleep stages slightly. These hypnotics are not as dose-dependent as the benzodiazepines, which means that there is a correct dose for adults and a correct dose for older people and doubling it does not increase their efficacy. Because of this, dependency is unlikely to develop and so far there has been no evidence of addicts using either of these medicines to overdose with. As with all new medicines, it takes time to be sure that there are no serious side effects, but at present these two new drugs seem to offer a quick way to get to sleep, overriding any preventive cause. In my opinion they are as close as you will get to an ideal sleeping pill until research discovers the brain substances that switch on your sleep centres.

This will not be long in coming. Already one has been isolated. Melatonin is secreted by your pineal gland which lies deep in the inter-brain. Melatonin decreases your core body temperature and increases sleepiness: in fact it puts you ready to go to sleep and has been used with success to help shift workers adjust to new shifts and to allow the blind to get a regular sleep pattern. It will be followed, I am sure, by further natural products that will enhance sleep onset and maintenance. So far in Britain melatonin is only available on prescription on a named-patient basis but it is already on sale abroad. Although it is a natural product it may have serious side effects and I would not experiment with it until full testing has proved its safety.

This chapter has not been written to allow you to become a do-it-yourself doctor. It is merely to alert you to be aware that insomnia may not be just due to stress. If you have started to sleep less well and are not aware of the cause, seek a doctor's opinion to exclude organic disease. Even if you think your sleeplessness is due to stress, if it persists despite your efforts let your doctor give you a second opinion.

Summary

Never play cards with any man called 'Doc'.
Never eat at any place called 'Mom's'. And
never, ever, no matter what else you do in
your whole life, never sleep with anyone
whose troubles are worse than your own.

Nelson Algren

1. Insomnia is not an illness. It is a symptom
which may accompany an illness.

2. If you suddenly find you are sleeping less
well and the condition does not clear up in a
couple of weeks, you should get a check-up
from your doctor.

3. If you have a chronic disease, the onset of
insomnia may mean that the condition is
becoming poorly controlled and needs reassessment, perhaps urgently.

4. Hypnotic medication should be short-acting,
have no effect on your sleep pattern and only be
taken for a short time until the underlying cause
has been found and treated.

5. Even if you have chronic ill health, your
sleep may be improved by a good pre-sleep

routine. A comfortable day usually follows a good sleep.

Case History 1

She was tall, slim and rather depressed when I saw her first. In her late thirties, she had slept poorly all her life, especially at times of stress. Her problem at present was that she was waking at four in the morning and then felt unable to get to sleep. She had been diagnosed as being mildly depressed, but treatment of this had not helped. The medication merely made her feel exhausted all day, so she had stopped it.

I asked her what she thought was the cause and she told me that she had done a spell as a shift worker, starting at four in the morning, and she thought she was reverting to that pattern for no reason.

I examined her, finding a scar on her abdomen but little else. Blood results were all normal, she assured me. Her doctor had done them recently. Had he checked her urine and her thyroid function? He had, and they were also normal. This seemed to rule out organic disease. I inquired about the scar.

She had had Crohn's Disease when she was younger and had had most of her large bowel removed. The scar was from a temporary

37

colostomy. If I had not seen it I might not have asked about her alimentary tract. She had long since forgotten the episode. She told me she had felt well, lived a normal life and ate a good, balanced diet.

There seemed few clues so far and I was half-inclined to accept her theory of why she did not sleep. However, I persisted and got a story of poor sleep all week but better sleep at the weekend. Her own doctor had thought that the stress of her job was keeping her awake through the week, but when she relaxed at the weekend she slept.

She did not agree with him. She said she could cope with her job and enjoyed it. She suggested that she would enjoy it more if I could find her a decent night's sleep.

We both decided against a trial of sleeping pills, she because she had tried them and they had not worked, and I because short-term help was not what she needed.

I continued to ask about her weekends, because if she slept better then she must be doing something right. She told me she went out to dinner every Saturday.

When was her last meal?

Nine or ten at the weekends, she told me.

What about the other meals?

At the weekend she had a decent breakfast and a cooked lunch. She then admitted that during the week she usually missed breakfast, ate sandwiches for lunch and had high tea so that she could watch television and finish any work from the day. Without most of her large bowel she would not absorb nourishment as easily as other people. I began to wonder if she was waking hungry.

When I suggested this to her she was interested. We devised a daily food intake schedule that she could cope with which included a large slice of fruit cake and a hot milk drink last thing at night. With this she slept through, just as she often did at weekends after a late dinner.

It is easy to diagnose stress where a patient has a stressful job, but if it persists it should be investigated fully.

Case History 2

'Ever since I got the central heating I have slept badly,' he said.

I had known Clive for some years. He seldom came to surgery, but his mother used to tell me how well he was doing. 'Clive is in the works' football team; Clive is getting a promotion; Clive has got married and has got a new house.'

'Is your bedroom too hot?' I asked.

'No, we keep the heating off there,' he answered, 'but I wake dry and then I feel I have to pass urine. It is very disruptive and means I'm tired at work.'

I agreed with him. Continuously getting up at night presages a long day.

'Nothing worrying you?' I asked.

'Not really. Of course the mortgage is bigger than we expected, but I can manage. I'm not a worrying type.'

'Then I think I should give you a full examination and see what we find,' I said.

It did not surprise me when I found his urine showed very positive for sugar. Clive had diabetes. His thirst and frequent need to pass urine were strong pointers to the condition. He had not noticed them through the day because he was busy.

He had to take insulin, but very quickly became used to balancing his blood sugar and seemed unfussed by this new development. His uncle had well-controlled diabetes and was a great help with advice and support in the early stages.

Clive told me the nicest thing about it all was that once his treatment had been settled his sleep pattern returned and he was as full of bounce as usual all day.

Chapter Three

The long-term causes
of stress insomnia

'I'm tired. I go to bed and then the thoughts come. They don't let me get to sleep.'

Don't you just know that feeling?

Stress, and the anxiety that it causes, is the main cause of insomnia in the western world. Of all those people who come to their doctors complaining that they can't get to sleep, for 80 per cent the cause is anxiety.

Most of you are aware of the problem but are powerless to prevent the worrying thoughts that chase round and round in your mind like rats in a trap, putting your body into a 'flight or fight reaction', leaving your brains hot and sore and completely destroying anything but the most transitory sleep.

Some of you are chronic worriers. You learned to rabbit on in your mind about quite minor matters in youth. The habit is often inherited. Patients have said to me that they feel

41

secure when they have a nice minor worry to nag away at. If they have none, they feel at a loss. After some years of this sort of practice you begin to find that the stabilizing worries of daytime spill over to disturb your sleep. Later on you get into bed and shut your eyes and the worry worked on through the day still dominates your thinking and holds your mind captive. Even if you do manage to fall asleep, you wake early and steeply right into the same worry as if it had been waiting.

Stress is caused by many things, but basically is your perception of overwhelming difficulty and your perception of your inability to cope with this perceived problem. Let me explain with a case history.

A patient of mine is a musician. He got a threatening letter from another musician with whom he had played for some time in a casual way. They had drifted apart amicably enough, but when my patient started to become well known from his playing with another accompanist, his first partner wrote to say that he should be compensated financially for the split as this fame had been built on the original duo's work. My patient was very upset by this letter. He felt threatened and feared a miserable time being hauled through the courts, paying for lawyers, perhaps being found liable for payment which he could ill afford. The hostility of the letter was a surprise. He explained that the writer had been a friend. They had had a beer together; they had rehearsed together; they had done a few gigs. The arrangement was mutually beneficial in that they had got a bit of extra money as a casual duo playing in hotels. It had stopped when his ex-friend had moved to another town and had not suggested coming back to continue the duo. My patient could think of nothing he had said or done to suggest that his first duo was a partnership. All night he found himself going over and over their time together and worrying about what would happen.

His perception of the problem had blown up out of all proportion. I asked him to tell me the actual problem. When he thought about this he said, 'He may envy my present success, which has been built since we parted and is due mostly to my new accompanist, who knows a lot of people who need a duo. He does not have any rights to our present income. If he goes to law I shall go to my own union, which has a legal department so I shall not be out of pocket.'

'So why are you worrying?'

'I tend to worry about things,' he confessed, 'and especially at night when I am not thinking of other things. Thinking about it as you have made me do makes me realize I do not really have a problem and I have a great sense of relief. I shall sleep well tonight.'

His perception of the problem had been blown out of all proportion to the actual difficulty. In his case, the actual difficulty was non-existent. It is not always so, but it is essential to get past the perceived problem to the true problem. Some of us are promoted beyond our capability and cannot cope; some are trying to do more than they reasonably can; some find their home or job responsibilities more than they can accept. They should take time to discuss these problems with their partners, a sensible friend or a trained counsellor, get down to the actual problem from the perceived and then make a decision about how to cope with it.

My patient's decision was to write to his ex-accompanist and tell him firmly that their casual arrangement had no rights on either side and had been terminated by his friend when he moved away. He went on to say that he was sending a copy of his letter to his union legal department. He did not hear from his ex-accompanist again and he became aware that when he found a worry obtruding into his sleep period he should at once work past the perceived problem to the actual and find an answer to that.

I have coined the term, 'The Scott "Sod it"

Technique' for actual problems. If there is nothing you can do to bridge the gap between what you should be doing and what you are doing, then it ceases to be your problem. You say 'Sod it', do what you can, stop agonizing about not coping, and allow someone else to find the solution. This is amazingly successful in relaxing stress. It may mean changing jobs and home responsibilities; it may require sensitive negotiation; but if your mechanism cannot cope, there is no point in trying to make it do so. That way lies heart attack and depression.

How does this technique help you with all the various forms of stress that home in at night to keep you awake?

Many patients come to me complaining of marital difficulties which they worry on about when they are in bed. Sleep is impossible. They seek oblivion and usually have come to surgery to ask for a sleeping pill. This is the worst possible treatment, as it merely shelves the problem until the next day, when it seems even more enormous.

What problem?

Sometimes their partners have gone off with someone else. Often this comes as a complete surprise to a spouse, who has felt secure and has been content with his or her present relationship. In this case they lie awake worrying about being left alone or with dependent children.

45

They feel enormous resentment and anger against the new partner and a feeling of betrayal against their own spouse. Financial insecurity and worry about the extra work caring for their children by themselves add to the fire in their brain that rages night after night as they lie in bed. By day they can verbalize their misery to others; by night it is turned inward.

'Why did he or she do this? I have done nothing to deserve it. Let them cope with the children. I will be lost without the children. How can I live? Who will pay? How I hate her/him. Can my partner not just forget that interloper and come back and make it all like it was before?'

This last is probably the most unlikely outcome. Whether there is reconciliation or not, nothing will ever be the same again. Trust has vanished. Complacency has gone. It is time to look beyond the huge perceptual difficulties to reality.

First, there is always the other side of perceived truth. Settled relationships do not break without dissatisfaction on at least one side.

'I have done nothing to deserve this' is never true and the first thing to find out is what caused the split. Levelling blame is counterproductive. It may be that complacency, boredom or disinterest all played their part. It is worth finding out the motivation for the defection so that if reconciliation takes place the same situation will not be allowed to develop. So often 'being in love' obscures your actual relationship.

There is no use lying thinking about the 'might have been'. You should accept the situation; say to yourself, 'Stop lying here resenting and hating and being afraid. Sleep loss will just compound this life crisis.' Through the day find out the reasons for the defection. A departing spouse is all too ready to tell. Accept these. They may be irremediable but they usually are worth paying attention to in any future relationship. Accept them as a lesson to be learned, not a fault. Clear your mind of guilt. Then go to a specialist to find out exactly how you stand financially. This is usually a lawyer or an accountant and he or she will be able to offer you clear paths from which to choose. Mobilize your support amongst family and friends, not by ranting on about your feelings but by asking how much help they are willing to offer. You will be surprised both ways.

At this point you enter the evening without guilt, resentment, hate and fear. When you go to bed you may be a little excited, but looking forward. You may have nostalgia for the past, but the acceptance that it has gone will not stand between you and sleep. It is wishing it back that keeps you awake.

The perceptual mountain of loss and difficulty has given way to acceptance of change. You can say, 'Sod them. They have the problem. I have a good lawyer and good friends and there may be good days ahead that I am now free to enjoy.' If you can say that last thing at night you will find no trouble falling asleep.

Family problems are the same. Lie awake worrying about the children and sleep will not come. Spend the day making clear decisions that satisfy the needs of both parents and children, negotiate a satisfactory settlement and the perceptual barriers and unknown horrors disappear.

It is the same for spouses facing violent, or drug-taking, or alcoholic partners. Worrying all night only compounds the problem. You may have to accept that your passive acceptance is not helping anyone. You may have to make a clear decision on whether it is your desire to put up with the problem or bale out and again, once the perceptual mountain of 'He/she cannot do without me', or 'What would I do on my own' has been thought through and expert advice has been listened to, the way ahead becomes obvious. Feelings change from worry to grief followed by acceptance, but the last of these does not cause insomnia.

Financial worries are the same. There is no use sitting worrying on a tipping gang plank. You may have to step off into unknown waters, but with expert advice you can do so with confidence. So much of sleep difficulty lies in scrabbling in your mind to keep things as they were. Life is not like that. Assertiveness training, supportive groups, counselling and expert advice are now available either free or at affordable cost. It is never fun changing your life, but if you sleep soundly the new day is a great deal better than if you don't.

Work stress may be treated in the same way. If you are trying to do more than you are able, stop. Say, 'Sod it.' Do what you can as well as you can. Leave someone else to do the rest. A reasonable firm will not penalize you. That is your misperception. They will adjust. If they do not, the actual problem remains. You cannot do all they ask so you may have to change your job and your lifestyle. Better that than the malaise that chronic insomnia brings.

Grief from bereavement is a special case in which I do often prescribe a short course of short-acting sleeping pills. Here the shock of loss is sometimes so great that for a day or two a brief, guaranteed oblivion can allow the first acceptance of change of circumstance and the healing that goes on in sleep is sometimes necessary for this. I use hypnotics that do not affect the sleep pattern so that healing may occur without habituation.

If you can diffuse these stresses that wear you out all night and prevent the restoration of body and mind that sleep brings, you will save yourselves a lot of ill health.

Chronic stress has been shown to have an effect on the body's immune system, reducing the white cells that protect from infection. Chronic stress predisposes you to infection; it has recently been found to have an association with an increased susceptibility to cancer. Stress overcomes the normal circadian rhythm of corticotrophin (ACTH) production from the pituitary gland, that great conductor of the hormonal orchestra of the body. Usually it peaks in the morning, stimulating the adrenal glands to give you a bit of a cortisol- and prolactin-rich boost at the start of the day. These levels remain high all day in response to chronic stress and may lead to hypertension, heart disease, impotence and loss of sex drive. It just makes you a little more likely to die before your unstressed colleagues.

Shrug it off if you like as just a statistic, but continuing to live with anxiety is a lot less pleasant than an unstressed day and a good night's sleep.

Getting past the perceptual problem to the

actual is the essential treatment of stress, but to do this you may need to escape the feeling of panic that is often associated with even thinking about the subject you are in thrall to. You also need to have some core strategy to remain stress free so that your perception of the ordinary difficulties of the day is not allowed to get out of hand and build a prison of anxiety that holds you awake at night.

If you have a religious belief you should use that to do this job and to strengthen your peace of mind. I grew up in the Christian tradition so it is easier for me to discuss it. 'Watch and Pray' instructs the New Testament and this is the essential way to gain 'the peace of mind that passeth all understanding'. Those of you who have managed to empty your minds of all except your search for God, who have offered your prayers for help for yourselves and others, for enlightenment, for faith, for courage to endure the future and accept death, for guidance in behaviour and relief of life's burdens, do gain that inner quiet that resolves stress. This is a lifetime's continuing pursuit, not a night-time panacea. To be effective it should be part of your daily lives and you should set a quiet time aside for the exercise.

I cannot claim to be other than a bit of a backslider, but when I have conformed I have

received great benefit and I do know that those
who are devout get enormous relief of stress and
an ability to accept actual situations. All religions have this offer of inner peace if you will
believe. Most people have their roots in some
religion, although they have grown too worldly
to believe or too busy to give the time to pray. If
the stresses of the world have begun to get on
top of you, it might be easier for you to return
to your childhood faith, be it Christianity,
Judaism, Bhuddism or Islam, and make it work
for you rather than to turn to new paths looking
for that peace of mind you had in youth.

Yoga, however, is popular at present and
many people use its exercises, both mental and
physical, to keep themselves stress-free. Yoga is
one of the six systems of Indian philosophy and
is based on the theory that you have a divine
potency, the Kundalini, at the base of your spine
which, if you are to reach the salvation of unity
within yourself and the universe, must be raised
through the vein, Sushumna, which runs the
length of your backbone via six Chakra
(wheels or psychic centres) to unite with your
centre of psychic power, the Sahasrara, at the
top of your head. This centre is often depicted
as a lotus with a thousand petals. Known in the
middle ages as Raja Yoga, Yoga has changed
and diversified to satisfy the needs and abilities

of many different people. In its purest form it requires intense development of the will using stretching exercises, meditation and mantra repetition until control of autonomic body functions, like heart beat and breathing, are attained. Hatha Yoga, the usual form of Yoga practised in the West, specializes in physical exercise to concentrate the mind and relax the body. It uses mantras to allow the mind to concentrate its energy on achieving unity of body, mind and universe. This way stress is eliminated from the body and many people find that they enjoy Yogic exercises and the relaxation of mind they bring, without delving too deeply into the religious purpose. The exercises are usually offered in a class by a trained teacher. This is quite sensible, as some of the exercises are complicated and take some months to master, as well as being strenuous. A trained teacher may advise which exercises are suitable for you.

Transcendental Meditation (T.M.) is another way of relieving stress. Its essentials may be taught in four two-hour lessons over four consecutive days or in a more leisurely fashion if desired. It is again taught by qualified T.M. practitioners. In the centre I went to, the lessons were not inexpensive.

Transcendental Meditation is a technique to

allow your thoughts to settle down until you reach complete mental quietness. Your body relaxes, stress disappears and for a while you feel great peace.

In India, about 1955, the Maharishi Mahesh Yogi began teaching this method of gaining inner peace. Before that he had spent years learning from the sage Guru Dev Bramananda Sarasawati. Following the death of Guru Dev, he spent two years in solitude from which he emerged to teach meditation. T.M. has become popular worldwide, which has to mean that it has some success in offering peace of mind.

During T.M. you follow a thought quietly into your mind until it fills the mind and then eddies forth, leaving you peacefully empty within your mind, waiting for the higher, fuller, feelings of completeness that you begin to experience. T.M. followers are given a meaningless mantra to lead them to this mental peace. They feel the choice of it is important and will make the experience one of increasing peace of mind if it is correctly chosen. They say you need a teacher. It may be so, but it is possible to achieve a degree of peace of mind by using some meaningless mantra from a Yoga book that makes you feel good when you repeat it, or just focusing your thoughts on a spot somewhere between your eyebrows and trying to empty your brain of thought. You are, in fact, reaching for stage 1 sleep. Thoughts may come and go. You should allow them to. You should not follow them. You should feel the comfort of your position. Think of some thing or place that you love and enjoy that feeling and let it go too. Soon, if you are sitting comfortably and your mind is quiet, you will feel a great sense of release. Twenty minutes of this a day is very therapeutic.

How far Transcendental Meditation will lead you towards enlightenment is something I cannot predict. I do know that being able to visit a quiet place in your mind is restful and will diffuse stress. Stage 1 and stage 2 sleep may well have stress-relieving effects and their preponderance towards the end of the night may not be just filling in time till you wake, but relieving the remembered stresses that your REM sleep has not managed to ameliorate.

The Alexander Technique is another method of relaxation for mind and body. Pioneered by the Australian actor F. Matthias Alexander (1869–1955) it has swept the world. He found that his voice became strangled if he stood with his chin up and his throat in a strained position. From this discovery he went on to find the most relaxed way to stand, sit and move. One of his exercises may be used to relieve stress.

Lie on your back on a comfortable flat surface, bend your knees up so that your back muscles relax and put a book under your head. Relax each muscle using a relaxation technique such as I have described in the next chapter. When your muscles lie very relaxed, so that you feel almost part of the ground beneath you, let your thoughts wander in a pleasant place or think of some happy event. Alexander Technique therapists aid relaxation by helping to stretch your back, but this is not necessary for the mental relaxation that you feel.

If all you need is time out of time, then these techniques are for you. They do not address any real problem. They do not produce any real answers. They do, however, give blessed relief from anxiety build-up and this may be enough for some people to continue their stress-filled life.

It is better, however, to address the problem, think it through and find a solution so that stress and anxiety have no place in your daily work other than to give you a bit of excitement and encouragement.

While these techniques may keep you going through the day so that your nightly stress build-up is minimalized you may need first-aid techniques to use if you still find sleep elusive. You may also need methods to help you get back to sleep if you have wakened during the night. These are in the next chapter.

Summary

Midnight shakes the memory
As a madman shakes a dead geranium
T.S. Eliot

Put your shoes at the door, prepare for life
T.S. Eliot

1. Different ways to achieve peace of mind and combat stress build-up are sprouting everywhere. Some are expensive.

2. These methods allow your mind 'time out of time', which eases the daily stress build-up of modern life.

3. These techniques do not solve your stress problems.

4. You must do this by looking past your perceived difficulty and your perceived inability to deal with it to the actual difficulty.

5. You must then make a decision to do

57

something about the actual difficulty.

6. This may entail a change in your lifestyle.

Case History

I came to treat Mr Jones through his wife. She
attended me with a tangle of minor complaints
which I gradually unravelled with her, finding a
deep anxiety that her marriage was falling
apart. Ever since her husband had been promoted he had changed towards her and the
children. Nothing was right. He shouted at the
children. He was becoming impossible to live
with. They all dreaded him coming home from
work.

'He didn't ever behave this way before,' she
wept. 'I think he must be having an affair or
something. He never comes home early like he
used to do.'

I suggested she might like to ask her husband
to come to me for a routine check-up and was
quite surprised when he turned up. His problem
was unexpected. He was not getting enough
sleep. He told me about his promotion and the
stress it had brought into his life. He worked
later and later to try to cope, but when he went
home the worry was with him and all night he

tried to work things out. Far from having an affair, he was sleep deprived.

He explained that he was an accountant, and a good one. Promotion to head of department was satisfying recognition of this and taking over the accounts of the whole firm was a delight. Managing his department was a nightmare. He felt neither trained nor able to deal with it. It was not his scene. Night after night he lay and worried about his decisions of the day. Had he been fair? Had he done right? Would he manage to keep his job?

His perception of his problem was out of control.

'Could he delegate the personnel organization to someone else?' I asked.

It had never been done before. He thought his general manager might think him incompetent if he suggested it.

'Was there someone in his unit who could do that part of his job well?'

'Yes,' he said. 'My secretary was built in with the bricks. She knows how everything should work.'

We discussed the effects of sleep deprivation and he accepted that he was not in need of medication so much as a quiet mind. I did not see him again, nor did I see Mrs Jones. Six months later I was called in to see her son with chickenpox. As she saw me to the door she said,

'Everything is fine, you know. I was silly to think he was having an affair. He was just getting used to his new promotion. Now he does all the accounting in the office and Carol, his secretary, has been made personnel officer. He arranged it with the general manager just after he had seen you.'

Clearly he had looked through his perceived mountain of inability to cope. He had said, 'I cannot do personnel organization so "Sod it." It is up to the firm to find a solution.' Negotiation with his general manager had resulted, not in demotion but in being given more of the work he revelled in, in exchange for the chore he could not perform.

Chapter Four

First-aid stress
insomnia cures

Bad nights are not always caused by life-shatter-
ing problems. Most people live pretty normal
lives, but when they go to bed sleep comes late
and if they wake they do not sleep again but
toss and turn the rest of the night.

If this has happened to you it is because you
have built up stress from everyday living without noticing it and should not let it continue.

Getting rid of even this stress needs time and
perseverence. It takes rethinking your daily
tasks and it may need a complete new lifestyle
with a new approach to work. Is that why you
don't settle down to get rid of it? Because it is
hard work?

How does it creep up on you?'

Stress, any stress, is a normal body reaction to
an unforeseen situation. The perception of a
problem brings a flow of adrenalin to your
blood that makes you awake and ready for

action. At first this is transient, a pleasant feeling of get up and go to combat a new job, a sudden crisis at work, an emergency situation. If the stress is not too great, you enjoy the stimulus the adrenalin brings. The flight or fight reaction of ancestral man still operates in the jungle of business life or in the no-less stressful family environment.

The stimulus to respond to an emergency is passed up from the lower brain centres to the higher, where fast decisions for reaction are taken. Flood the cortical higher centres and they become overwhelmed. Decisions block one another and total stasis may result.

In maritime disasters, when the whistle gives five short blasts and one long and you are instructed to put on a coat and move calmly to your lifeboat station, the majority obey. However, sailors have found passengers who have retired to bed and seem unable to get up; they speak of passengers who refuse to leave without a favourite book or toothbrush. These people have been overwhelmed by the demand for action and their brains can't cope. 'I am not like that,' you say.

I used to think that too. Then I was going down to London for my daughter's wedding. Because she wanted it there, the bridal party all stayed at a hotel. I was worried about leaving my medical practice, worried that the arrangements made so far from home would all run smoothly, anxious as any mother that my daughter would be happy in this new life. Sleep came slowly and when the fire alarm went in the middle of the night I got up and went to the lift and pressed the button for down.

Every hotel has notices telling you not to do this. Every hotel has arrows pointing to fire stairs.

It was not until I was halfway down that I realized I was being very silly, pressed the button for the next floor, and got out. I then went downstairs, despite an almost overwhelming urge to return to my room to retrieve the wedding dress.

It was a false alarm. Regardless of that, I had acted inappropriately and endangered myself, all because my stress level had been overwhelming.

This is why cruise liners practise lifeboat drill and businesses, fire drill. Overwhelmed higher brain centres may not function but the organizations hope that a practised reaction will be automatically followed as it is masterminded by centres embedded in the lower brain.

Life is not a series of fire alarms, or is it?

Morning starts with the stress of wondering if the mail will be delivered before you have to go to work. You have to get ready in time to catch the right train or bus. You hope the traffic will not make you late. You get uptight about motorists cutting in to keep you back. By the time you reach work you may well have that buzzing feeling in the brain that means a high stress level. It does not take much in many professions and jobs to keep that stress going. Deadlines for journalists, surgeries and house calls for doctors, legal decisions for lawyers that have to be right. It extends to the factory floor and offices, where others may be able to work faster, where time-keeping is rigid but you want to get away to do something you think essential. Frustration and stress are now part and parcel of your daily life. Anxiety is the result. The thoughts that go round and round in your brain till it feels hot and sore are even more oppressive when you are trying to go to sleep and all other counter-stimuli, like television and conversation, have stopped. 'I should have said'; 'I should have done'; 'I should never have let them get away with ...' Round and round go your thoughts. You can't stop them. Sleep is a non-starter. The adrenalin pulsing in your bloodstream prevents any hope of rest.

You may drop off for a short time, but your sleep is fitful, never reaches those deep levels where growth hormone is released to repair the wear and tear of your body tissues and seldom gives your brain a chance to renew itself in dream sleep.

So much for stress at work. It is no less common at home. Mothers of young children are never free of the anxiety of wondering where their children are, what they are doing and if they need help. Many mothers adapt their sleep to remain in the lighter sleep planes so they wake easily if their children cry. They spend less time in deep, restorative sleep. This gradually has an effect on their body. They are chronically tired, too tired to stop being anxious. It becomes a habit and the habit prevents their getting to sleep, so a spiral develops of poor sleep followed by anxious days followed by even less sleep. In the West, mothers of young children who opt to stay at home to bring their family up are ghettoized for the first few years until they are able to attend a mother and toddler group and share conversation and problems with other mothers, hear their solutions, empathize with their feelings and become one of a group diffusing each other's tensions.

So if you recognize yourself in any of the scenarios I have described, what should you do about it?

Nothing beats facing up to the perceptual problem and your perceptual inadequacy to deal with it, accepting the actual problem (and actual inadequacy if there is any) and then changing the situation so that you can actually cope. In the short term, however, while you gear yourself up to what may be a complete change of lifestyle, you may need first-aid methods to nullify stress and worry that stops you getting to sleep and getting back to sleep if you wake in the middle of the night. You must learn to wind down in the evening and prepare for sleep to be able to take over your mind by reducing your mental alertness.

Set aside a time in the evening to be by yourself and consider which thoughts are going to trouble you that night. List the anxieties of the day. Write them down. Make a decision about each of them and write that down too. Even if your decision is that you can do nothing about the problem that night and will have to put off coping with it until the next day or the next week, when you will look at it again, your brain will accept this. Write the decision against each problem and keep it at your bedside. You can then comfort yourself that all your worries are dealt with for the night and you have no further need of thought. 'Thinking' is the enemy of sleep and at night must be avoided at all costs. Thinking is like alcohol to an alcoholic. Start the night with a problem to work out and you are heading for a 'white night'. Thought must be blocked to allow normal sleep to take over.

One way to do this is to repeat a meaningless word over and over quietly out loud or in your mind. Some psychologists suggest 'the' or 'and' repeated every couple of seconds. Yogic meditators use the words 'aum' or 'ram,' repeated in the same way to enable themselves to empty their minds of thought. They concentrate on the sound of the word and its shape and allow other thoughts to be blocked out. Yogic stretching and relaxing exercises learned at classes are also useful. One exercise I would like to mention is done in the Shavasana, or 'corpse' position.

Lie flat on your back, arms extended palms up and a little away from your side. Let your legs lie straight and relaxed, the feet slightly apart. Make sure there is no tension in your neck and that your head is in a comfortable position. Relax completely, trying to merge with the bed beneath. Relax each muscle group from your feet upwards. Take a deep breath and blow it out gently, then breathe quietly as you repeat, 'aum, aum', or 'ram, ram, ram' to yourself, filling your mind with the sound and blocking thought. As you slide into sleep you will probably turn into a more comfortable position in which to continue the night.

Transcendental meditators suggest that their meditation should take place in the daytime when full emptying of the mind can take place with the healing that accompanies it. They counsel against meditation in bed in case you fall asleep. It seems to me, therefore, that you can use T. M. as a hypnotic if it helps. Just lying quiet, concentrating on a spot between your eyebrows and allowing thought to empty from your brain until your whole head feels empty and quiet is a very relaxing exercise. Little thoughts may begin to seep in and out, inconsequential thoughts that have no power. Allow them to come and go. They are the herald of stage 1 sleep.

Another way to block thought is to listen to music. I have already described my series of cassettes of classical music played at the brain-wave rate as it slips into sleep. 'Sound Asleep for Babies', 'Sound Asleep for Adults' and 'Sound Asleep for Seniors' bludgeon thoughts and worries from the mind and sleep takes over. I find it a pleasant way to circumvent worry. Other people tell me they sometimes listen to the radio turned low or read a book. Reading last thing is a time-honoured way to get to sleep, but it should be approached with caution. If it helps, use it, but if it stimulates thought, it may be counter-productive.

It is as important to allow the body to unwind as it is to block thought. It is surprising how anxiety or worry causes tension in every muscle. Simple relaxation techniques abound and I shall start by describing one. Follow it completely to relax the whole body just before sleep or during the day if you want to 'crash out' for twenty minutes in a comfortable chair.

Some people enter their beds with a sense of failure. 'I'll never sleep tonight', and 'I'll be a wreck tomorrow if I can't get to sleep' is the thought in their heads. Never let this sort of thought persist. Challenge it with something much more positive like, 'Sleep will come in its own time if I continue to do my relaxation exercises or listen to my music.'

Relaxation Technique

1. Sit in a comfortable armchair that you can't fall off or lie comfortably in bed or on a thick carpet on the floor with a pillow under your head. Get into your usual position for going to sleep.

Stretch your left foot out and pull the toes up towards your shin, continue to stretch the calf muscles and tense the muscles in your thigh. Tense, tense, tense, for about 8 seconds, then relax the leg and foot completely. Let the leg fall slack. Feel it sink into the bed or onto the floor relaxed and heavy. Think into the relaxation and make the feeling familiar. Try to relax deeper and deeper. Take at least 15 seconds to do this.

2.   Repeat this for the other leg and foot.

3.   Now the stomach and buttock area. Take a deep breath in, using your diaphragm, that muscle that separates the chest from the abdomen and helps breathing, like a piston going up and down. You will feel it pushing the abdominal wall out as you breathe in. Put a hand on your upper abdomen if you are in doubt. You should feel it rise with inspiration. Tense your stomach muscles as if you were expecting a blow, now tense all the muscles round the hips and buttocks. Pull up your perineal muscles as if you were trying to stop yourself going to stool or passing urine. Pull, pull pull. Concentrate on the tension for 8 full seconds then breathe out and let the tension flow out of the muscles with expiration. Breathe away gently. Let the hard corset of contracted muscle go soft and heavy and sink into your bed or chair. Think into the relaxation, feel how the muscles should be when they are relaxed and try to increase that feeling of relaxation. Concentrate on the relaxation for about 15 seconds.

4.   Take another deep breath in, using all the muscles of your chest wall and the diaphragm, go on breathing in by lifting your shoulder muscles to give more room. Hold the tension for 8 seconds, shoulders back and taut, chest out,

diaphragm down. Then breathe out gently and let all those muscles relax. First feel those shoulders sag into jelly-like softness, the ribs relax and the diaphragm come up gently. Breathe away softly and continue to try to relax the shoulders further. This is a particularly important part of the body to relax. Much mental stress is reflected by tension in the shoulders. Later on, tense shoulder muscles will warn you that you are stressed and you will be able to diffuse the tension by taking a breath and relaxing the shoulder girdle without anyone noticing.

5. Now the neck. Press it back into the chair or into the bed, then relax it. Contract for 8 seconds, relax for 15 seconds and think into the relaxation to try to deepen it.

6. Facial tension is another major sign of stress. Tense jaws that grind at night, stressed muscles round the eyes, braced against a tension headache. You all know these miseries without realizing they are just your body's way of showing you that your brain is overloaded. Tense up the jaws, scrunch up the muscles round the eyes, frown and pull the sides of your mouth out towards your ears in a grimace. You may not look a pretty sight but hold the tension for 8 seconds and then let it go. Feel the relief as

your jaw hangs down, relaxed; your lips fall in; your eyes lie quiet and your brow becomes unlined. Let your eyes close gently and enter the dark, comfortable feeling of total relaxation.

7. Go back round your body in your mind, concentrating on tensing and re-relaxing any muscular area that has become tense. Breathe gently and comfortably, feel yourself sink into the comfort of your bed or chair.

Now let your mind wander over some pleasant place. Is it the golf course where you imagine yourself teeing off and playing each hole? Is it a garden remembered from youth? Is it a story that you tell yourself, or a comforting bit of poetry?

If you are in bed, you can use music or any of the thought-blocking techniques I have described to occupy your mind. Feel cool peace of mind and concentrate on keeping it. Relax all over and allow the brain to take you in to sleep. The tired brain is only too willing to offer the healing processes of sleep if you will allow it to by stopping the adrenalin flow of anxiety.

Some insomniacs find they get to sleep by trying to stay wakeful while lying very relaxed. Their concentration blocks anxiety and enables sleep.

Keeping the thoughts that wake you out of your mind is the essential step. For people whose thoughts keep them awake, a good sleep hygiene habit that does not vary, followed by some of the techniques I have listed above, should help.

Massage, reflexology, aromatherapy may all be added to a basic sleep hygiene habit and will be described later; as will the methods of other systems of medicine.

All these techniques may be used to get you back to sleep if you wake through the night. The essential thing here is not to let your brain start to think. Keep it empty of all but fleeting thoughts. One patient told me she used to go to the bathroom without putting on the light and very often without opening her eyes. This may not be possible in all houses, but the less you allow yourself to wake the easier it is to return to sleep. If you cannot sleep again within reasonable time and become restless, it is probably sensible to get up and have a warm milk or barley water drink and read till you are tired and then restart your routine of preparing to sleep. Anything is better than thrashing round the bed unable to get back to sleep. The problem with rewakening and retrying to get back to sleep is that time passes and you may become seriously deprived of sleep if you have to do it too often. Lying quietly, allowing body relaxation and using your thought-blocking techniques, will enable more stage 1 and 2 sleep to occur than you think and may be the better way.

A more rigorous technique for dealing with insomnia is to keep a sleep diary for two weeks, totting up the number of hours that you actually sleep. Calculate your average sleep time for these nights. Go to bed so that you will have only that amount of sleep time before your alarm wakes you at your regular morning wake-up time. This prevents you thrashing around in bed, sleepless. It also stops you trying to make up sleep and lying wakeful in bed for longer and longer periods. As you get into the habit of going to bed and going to sleep you may begin to go to bed a quarter of an hour earlier week by week until you find that you again cannot sleep through the whole night. If you feel well rested by day, this may be all the sleep time you need.

Summary

Sleep is when all the unsorted stuff comes flying out as from a dustbin upset in a high wind.

William Golding

1. To get sound sleep, anxieties from the day must be listed and a decision made about them

so that they no longer obtrude into your mind at night.

2. Thought is the enemy of sleep. It must be blocked.

3. Relaxation techniques may help you get to sleep and get back to sleep if you wake in the night.

4. These are first-aid measures. In the end, the original stress or anxiety causing insomnia must be faced and diffused.

Case History 1

Jean was at university. Her final exams were coming up at the end of term and she wanted to do well. She was not anxious about her exam. She told me she had prepared well for it; her previous results were all good and though she was excited she was not nervous, yet.

'The week before the exams I will sleep less well,' she told me. 'I did the same at school every year, but I soon make it up afterwards. I find it hard to get to sleep, but once I am over I sleep all night.'

This time she was finding it hard to get off, then waking after a couple of hours and finding a return to sleep impossible. Her mother had always found sleep difficult, she told me. They were both natural worriers.

Jean's mother had newly been diagnosed as having an overactive thyroid gland and was undergoing treatment. Jean's boyfriend of three years had suddenly become cool. Their settled relationship was in jeopardy. They were both graduating at the end of term and he had started discussing the idea of a separation for his first year after university to see if the relationship would hold. She was an only child from a one-parent family and she and her mother were close.

She said that she had always kept a set routine before bed. It helped her get to sleep. She was tired at the end of the day and though she tossed and turned a bit, she got off to sleep but wakened worrying about little things that she might or might not have done the previous day. If she dozed off, it was just for an hour or so. She was becoming very tired.

Although young, Jean impressed me by having a lot of insight into her problems. She readily accepted that she needed a stable background to function well. I asked her if she was afraid that she was also hyperthyroid and she confessed that her mother's first symptoms of the condition had been sleep disturbance. Complete blood tests allayed that fear. Jean appeared very healthy. We talked about her inner security and she admitted that with both her boyfriend and mother not providing back-up she was quite nervous when she thought about being left on her own. Her future sud-denly seemed rather frightening.

I suggested to her that this was probably her main anxiety and had so filled her mind that all the normal worries of the day, which she would have taken in her stride if she had been secure, now troubled her. We decided that she would have to work out a strategy for her life, with and without the boyfriend, that would keep her feeling secure. In the short term, because she loved classical music, she was going to use 'Sound Asleep for Adults' to help her to sleep. She would add it in to her bedtime routine, switch off her light and switch on the music, concentrate on it and allow it to take her into sleep. Before she went to bed she was going to make a list of all the little worries she thought would annoy her through the night, write a decision against them and then if they surfaced, tell herself that she had thought about that worry and the decision was made.

She rang after a week to tell me that her sleep had improved. She got to sleep quicker and woke less often. She was trying to get together a life plan that she could follow after university even if she was on her own and had started going to a Scottish country dance society once a week, which she enjoyed and which allowed her to meet new friends.

In six weeks she came to see me again. Her sleep was now back to normal. Her mother had finished treatment and felt a lot better.

'What about the boyfriend?' I asked.

She blushed and held out her left hand, which now had a ring on the fourth finger. They were going to get married after they qualified she said.

She had diffused her anxieties, not by facing up to possible loss but by having her personal security reformed round her. Her small daily worries had been dealt with by my first-aid techniques. She might face the same sleep loss if she met another situation in which people on whom she depended for support reneged on her.

Case History 2

Mrs Mains was thirty-five, thin, grey-faced and miserable. When I saw her first I sympathized with her doctor for having given her a course of antidepressants. I would have been tempted to myself, except that she told me at once that they had done no good; they hadn't even helped her get to sleep.

Her main problem was worrying at night. She

got into bed and started to worry, which stopped her sleeping. When she did get off, she woke early and straight into the same worry as if she had never stopped. She was now tired all day, depressed and weepy.

What had happened in her life to cause all this?

She knew that too. Her husband had gone off with his secretary, leaving her in a big empty house with one child who was still at school. She felt tied to the house because she did not want to disrupt her son's education.

'How could he do it to me?' she wailed. 'I was a good wife. I looked after him, and all the time he was going out with her in the shirts I had ironed and the shoes I had polished. I lie in bed and I can't stand it. I want to hurt them both.'

Beside her resentment was fear of what would happen to her and her son.

'I can't keep that huge house and pay the rates. I don't know what to do.'

I told her she must think past her perception of enormous difficulty, and she was a great deal calmer after she had seen her lawyer and got her financial position straight. She still was not sleeping. Together we went over her feelings for her husband, his new partner and her own part in the separation. She began to see that she had, in fact, been growing away from her husband for some years. They had little in common and had seldom gone out together. Without guilt she began to look at the problem in a different light

Every night she made a list of the worries she knew would keep her awake and made decisions on them. She took up Yoga and went to an exercise class when her son was at school. She also began going back to church and found the young wives' group there supportive.

After a month of these activities she came to see me looking a much better colour. She even smiled.

'Last night in my decisions session I decided to make the house work for me,' she said. 'I am going to start doing bed and breakfasts.'

'Great idea,' I enthused.

'Better than that. I slept well for the first time.'

I saw her in the street six months later. 'How is it going?'

'I'm full for the next six months. Couldn't be better. We'll have enough money for a holiday soon.'

'But how is your sleep?'

'Oh, that's fine now. I'm too tired at the end of the day to do other than get into bed and put out the light. Morning comes much too soon.'

Real tiredness from real exercise encourages sleep. She had worked out her actual problem and was coping well.

Chapter Five

Herbal remedies, aromatherapy and reflexology

Herbalism

Since we started eating plants we have known that some make us feel different. Those who listed these effects and used the plants to treat others became the first herbalists and in writing their experiences down they produced the first herbals. Imhotep, priest-physician in Egypt about 2980 BC, architect of the Step Pyramid of Sakkara, acquired such a reputation for his cures that he was made a demigod. Later, the Ptolomies named him God of Medicine and he was worshipped in temples and shrines all over Egypt and Nubia.

Galen, Greek physician, herbalist and philosopher, lived about AD 130–200, and with Hippocrates founded the Western tradition of allopathic medicine, in which doctors see disease as an invasion to be repulsed. Treatment is directed at attacking the invader. This is not the same in the East. Chinese physicians, as you will see later in the book, consider that an imbalance in your body has allowed the illness to take hold and treatment is directed at restoring your body balance so that you can attack the invading disease yourself.

As the two traditions come closer together, Western doctors offer a more holistic approach. They now try to treat the whole patient and support him while still looking for and isolating an invading organism to conquer. In this endeavour, many doctors look to old treatments such as herbs, massage and aromatherapy. They feel that these have wider effects on their patients and may support the whole body while they also offer a specific drug to cure a disease.

In fact, herbs may have a profound effect. Taken internally, they are a strong medicine. Doctors now look back to the writings of physicians like Galen to see if there are herbs that they have forgotten which may be of use.

One source of Galen's comments on the properties of herbs can be found in William Turner's herbal, published in 1551. Turner was Dean of Wells and physician to the Duke of Somerset. His herbal, written so long ago, has the accurate observation of any modern medical tome.

In many ancient herbals, insomnia and its

treatment play little part. It was not thought to be a serious problem. 'The flux' and 'stoppage of the water' and 'the gout' get far more attention and cures listed. You begin to think that insomnia is a modern disease. It is not. People did not always sleep well in 1551 either. William Turner was well aware of it and describes the various causes of sleep loss very accurately.

He writes, 'Oftimes a man cannot sleep by reason of the heat of the brains moving . . .' or when melancholy is risen into the head, sometimes commeth it by reason of exceeding heat.' He records that sweet almonds 'make one sleep pleasantly' and also recommends lettuce leaves, lettuce seed, violet leaves, barley water and cream or pottage of peas taken late in the evening.

The sap of poppies has always been known to produce sleep and Turner was aware of this. Extracts of poppies are opiates and they are now legally controlled as medication because of their addictive properties. Opiates are only available on prescription from a doctor, so are no longer herbal remedies available to the general public over the counter. Poppy seed has not the same effect, and is sold as decoration for bread and cakes.

The greatest early herbal, the *Codex Vindobonensis*, was written in the sixth century by

Pedianos Dioskurides, probably a Greek arm
doctor and a contemporary of Pliny. Thi
handwritten manuscript describes how an
when to gather plants and recommends an
herbalist to know plants in all their stages o
growth. His precepts hold good today, and ma
be said to be the origin of the science of Botany

Throughout Europe herbals continued to b
written. During the middle ages the drawing
tended to be stylized and not easy to recognize
but gradually naturalism prevailed and by th
time printing came into its own to allow man
copies to be circulated, first in woodcut an
then as metal-engraved etchings, pictures c
plants became easily identifiable. Great name
abound. Some, like Thomas Culpepper, liste
plants with their medicinal properties; others
such as Elizabeth Blackwell, produced beautifu
etchings as well. Every housewife had her ow
herbal, either in her head or written down, t
deal with the minor illnesses with which she wa
faced. Getting the doctor was a costly busines:

By the eighteenth century doctors began t
use herbs less as 'cupping' and 'blood-letting
and metallic-based medicines such as mercuri
and arsenical compounds became popula
Herbal remedies were relegated to old wive
simples and the main herbal scientists took the
subject forward to become the science of Botan
rather than medicine.

At this time Westerners emigrating to America found that the Indian tribes still used plants as medicines and in many cases very skilfully. Settlers learned from the Indians and set out to sell these herbal cures to other settlers. Some of these 'White Indian Doctors' were charlatans but some, like Samuel Thomson (1769–1843), were skilled physicians. His book on herbal remedies was imported to Britain, where it became popular.

At this time the industrial revolution had forced many country people into towns, but they knew their plants and often tried to keep a little garden to remind themselves of their country origins. So herbalism began to flourish again. At the more educated level, Albert Coffin returned from America and his book, an adaptation of the Thomson original, was adopted as the text book of the new National Institute of Medical Herbalists, founded in 1864. Interestingly, one of its founding members was a Jesse Boot of Nottingham, who was also to found the great Boots chemist chain.

Herbal medicine has come a long way from those first practitioners, just as allopathic treatments have changed from the 'cupping' and arsenic and mercury powders of the past. Modern herbalists see their remedies as coming first in the allopathic chain of medical treatment. They support the idea of home remedies to see if some simple, easily available herbal medication can control a problem before it becomes necessary to go to the doctor to get a prescription that may also have strong side effects.

Medical herbalists are trained in all the medical sciences as well as in Botany and analytical techniques, but they prescribe only herbal remedies. They feel that your body, mind and spirit form a complex whole with constant corrective forces acting to maintain a healthy balance. To be effective, herbal remedies must strengthen these forces so their remedies, or 'simples' as they are called, may be a mixture of herbs with different actions to strengthen some forces and subdue others.

Just as Dioskurides recommended so many years ago, modern herbalists learn the character of the plants they use. They describe their properties as 'rising', 'floating', 'condensing' and 'sinking' and use plants taken at these times for different purposes. Rising and floating remedies will increase body heat and increase your resistance against invading pathogens and prevent sinking tendencies such as diarrhoea or prolapses. Astringents, emetics and expectorant mixtures are examples of these.

Sinking remedies reduce heat in your body and lower body activity. They include sedatives, bitters, antispasmodics, purges and diuretics and are used to counter vomiting, headaches, nervous dyspepsia and sleeplessness.

Herbal medicines, because of their low dosage, are slow to show an effect and therefore have to be taken for some time before their action becomes apparent. Sleeping potions are no different. However, herbal remedies may become addictive, just as the stronger synthetic drugs are. In addition, taking any herb for long periods may also have other effects on the body which may be harmful. This must always be taken into account with any long-term medication and the risks assessed and accepted. You do not know whether any substance you eat may cause cancer or inflammation of various organs. This is why a balanced varied diet is probably a safer one than one using a single product all the time.

The modern herbs to treat insomnia encourage your body to relax and so enable your normal sleep process to occur.

Valerian has been used as a sedative for many years. It is said to subdue nervous excitement and sleeplessness. Its effect may be enhanced by adding balm or lemon balm, which suppresses nervous excitment, or hops which check nervous sleeplessness. Herbalists prescribing for sleeplessness are trying to correct any imbalance in your body forces as well as offering you sedation. They may well use a mixture of herbs

87

to achieve that effect. For self-medication it is safer to use a single mild herb infusion that you know suits you and has few side effects. Valerian is quite a strong sedative and could become addictive if you take it regularly for any length of time. Hops may cause nausea and sweating in overdose, as well as having a slightly oestrogenic effect. Patients have told me that camomile and hibiscus infusions have brought them wild dreams, but this is not generally reported. Interestingly, both camomile and peppermint's main use is as a digestive tract settler and their sedative effects are secondary to this.

Oats and barley are good for insomnia. Consider a plate of porridge and milk for a late night supper.

Barley water is made by boiling two handfuls of barley in two litres of water until the barley is soft, then allowing it to cool. You may strain off the residue and store the barley water in your fridge, using it as necessary, hot or cold. Like many herbal remedies it does not keep for ever so needs to be made when you want it. A barley water drink of an evening is very soothing. An infusion made by pouring boiling water over a piece of bitter (Seville) orange peel is also said to be effective. Olives are also said to aid relaxation.

Oats, barley, lettuce, pea soup, olives, and orange peel tea can do no harm, but other herbal remedies such as passionflower, skullcap (*scutellaria laterifolia*), limeflower, valerian, verbena, hibiscus, hops, and lemon balm can make you unwell in overdose, so if you want to use them as a sedative follow the instructions on the packet exactly or ask a qualified herbalist to advise you. Anyone may become intolerant or allergic to herbal teas or medications so make sure they suit you before you use them just as you do with any food or drink.

Many of these herbs may be bought at the herbalist with instructions on how much to use to make a cup of herbal tea. If you gather your own herbs, make sure they are clean and grow in some unpolluted spot. They should be gathered in dry weather just before the plant is fully developed and after the morning dew has evaporated from the plant. Spread them to dry in a well-ventilated place and store them in airtight jars away from light. They should always smell and look fresh when you use them.

Infusions are made by pouring boiling water on the herb and allowing it to stand for five or ten minutes, just like making tea. A teaspoon of herbs to a mug of water is a rough guide to getting an effective infusion.

Decoctions are made by simmering the herbal substance in water for about fifteen minutes and then straining off the liquid. You are trying to achieve the same sort of strength as with the infusions, so you must allow for some evaporation by adding more water.

Tinctures tend to be stronger and are alcohol-based herbal mixtures. They are usually measured out in drops and taken with water or milk.

Compresses are made by soaking clean cloths in a hot herbal infusion or decoction and applying them to the affected area until they cool.

Poultices use fresh or dried herbs bruised and applied direct to the skin or laid between pieces of gauze. They are made more effective by having heat applied over them, such as a warm hot-water bottle.

Most people have long forgotten how to recognize herbs, how to preserve them and how to use them. It is worth taking a course in herbalism if you want to use your own herbal remedies. Nowadays, herbalists have all these substances in their shops and are very happy to advise you how to take them and how much to use. If you grow them in your garden a herbalist will be able to show you how to use the fresh herbs so that you do not make your mixtures too strong.

I suggest that if you turn to herbal medicine, you ask the experts before you dabble. Certainly, if you are pregnant or breast feeding a baby you should ask a doctor or herbalist before you take strong herbal medicines.

When sleep is hard to come by herbalists, like doctors, wonder if their client has an underlying depression or anxiety and may suggest St John's wort, a herbal antidepressant, to lighten the mood or rauwolfia (Indian Snake Root) as a tranquillizer for anxiety.

Here is a case where a herbal remedy can produce strong side effects. I first knew of rauwolfia as a prescribable drug for high blood pressure. It has fallen out of use as newer drugs emerged because it is less effective than the new, synthetic mixtures and has more serious side effects. The herbal strength to treat anxiety is very much less than the strength needed to treat high blood pressure but even so, this is not an impotent medication.

Traditionally, different communities use different herbal concoctions to induce relaxation. They are often open to abuse. Kawa-kawa is a Polynesian drink which is both intoxicating and sedative. Hashish is used by some nations as a relaxant. Hashish or marihuana is also able to produce hallucinations and restlessness and at present is illegal in Great Britain.

Alcoholic drinks are part of this scene. Wine, brandy, port and sherry from grapes; whisky from barley; vodka from potatoes, to name but a few, produce sedation and sometimes deep sleep. Their action, however, does not last. If you take a strong drink of alcohol you may fall asleep rapidly but you will wake early, often with a headache and nausea. This is a herbal remedy that should be used with caution. I do have older patients who tell me they have never taken a sleeping pill in their lives but do often have a glass of whisky or wine late at night to make them sleepy. At present medical knowledge suggests that a small amount of alcohol may dilate your blood vessels and so have a beneficial effect on the heart circulation in older people. It has been in use for so long that there has to be some usefulness in these various alcoholic drinks. Addiction is, however, very possible and a serious consequence and I would advise you not to use alcohol for insomnia unless in very small quantities and not as a regular soporific in case you are tempted to raise the dose. Because alcohol interacts and often potentiates many other medicines, it has to be taken with caution if you are taking any other drugs.

Nowadays herbalists seek to provide gentle medicines which have an effect over the long term. Their training to offer this service takes four years and names of qualified herbalists may be obtained from The National Institute of Medical Herbalists, 56 Long Brook Street, Exeter, Devon EX4 6AH.

Herbalists feel that in their consultations they

are able to give time for patients to talk about their problems. This knowledge allows a trained herbalist to make up a balanced 'simple' to heal the whole person. In a way, this approach is closer to the Eastern medical disciplines, where internal body balance is sought. Herbalists speak of the balanced treatment offered by giving a whole herb as opposed to an extract of it. Valerian, for instance, is a tranquilliser but has diuretic effects. Herbal medicine carries this natural balance further by bringing together different herbs to give a required overall effect. For sleep they might suggest a mixture of valerian and passionflower for sedation but balance it with damiana which supports the nervous system in a more stimulating way. This sort of mixture is beyond an amateur herbalist and you should not attempt it. There is no reason, however, why you should not try a cup of hot barley water with a twist of Seville orange peel in it to help you get to sleep.

There are many mixed herbal infusions, pre-packed and ready for use. They do not contain caffeine as do tea and coffee. Look for peppermint, passionflower, hibiscus, camomile, marjoram or lemon balm if you want a night-time drink that will help you get to sleep. Find the mixture that suits you best and keep it handy for a night when you think you need a little help 'getting over'. Never become dependent on even a herbal infusion for gaining sleep. Rather, treat the root cause.

Some people are unhappy about the mystique surrounding a doctor who offers a quick consultation and an unreadable prescription. Herbalists offer an alternative and feel that their training is adequate to allow them to refer their patient to an appropriate doctor or specialist if that is necessary. They are anxious to distance themselves from untrained herbalists who offer unsafe advice. If you like the idea of herbal medicine, find a qualified herbalist to consult.

Perhaps because taking unknown herbs inwardly can be alarming; perhaps because herbalists realize that many of their products could work as baths or when massaged into the skin with oil, aromatherapy has become very popular.

Aromatherapy

Aromatherapy has been around a long time. The Ancient Egyptians extracted the essential oils from plants and used them in perfumes, ointments and salves. Their expertise was so great that the dead bodies they mummified using salves and ointments from plant and mineral origins, are still in good condition today. We tend to credit the French chemist Gattefosse for the more recent research into the medicinal properties of essential oils in the 1920s, but aromatherapy was used by all the Eastern medical traditions over thousands of years and it may again be our interest in their techniques that brings it into prominence these days.

Essential oils are the essences extracted from flowers, leaves and other parts of trees and plants. The method of extraction varies according to what part of the plant is being extracted, but is usually some form of distillation. These essential oils are the basis of many perfumes, but for aromatherapy should be bought from a recognized herbalist or source that guarantees their natural orign. There are many cheaper, synthetic essences which are said not to be so effective.

Marjoram is a useful sedative and gives a warm relaxed feeling if used in a bath or as a massage. Geranium has an ameliorating effect on nervous tension while stimulating the skin circulation. Neroli is distilled from the white blossom of the bitter orange tree. It was used in Roman times as a treatment for insomnia and anxiety. Brought back into common use by Anna Maria Orsini, the Princess of Nerola, it now bears her name. Ylang ylang comes from a tropical flower grown in the Philippines, where they use its essential oil to relieve depression and insomnia. It mixes well with sandalwood or jasmine to give a very relaxing massage. Camomile essence is equally effective as a topical sedative. Lily of the valley may allay nervous palpitations; violet is said to alleviate melancholy; lavender and rose may be used to gain relaxation. They are all lovely scents.

Because the essential oils are so concentrated, they need to be mixed with an inert carrier oil to make a massage medium. Soya, almond or grapeseed oils are light carrier oils. Olive, avocado or wheatgerm oils are rather heavier and may leave a sticky feeling after a massage unless they have been diluted with one of the lighter oils. Use about five drops of essence to a large tablespoonful of base oil to make enough for a single massage. In a bath, five drops of essence is enough to give a scented, relaxing bath.

The chief places in your body where tension arises are in your shoulders and back. A warm massage of these areas using lavender or essence of rose diluted in vegetable oil is very helpful in relieving tension, and essence of violet encourages sedation.

As with all plant extracts, these essential oils

may cause skin irritation and an allergic reaction in some people, so it is wise to put a very small amount on the inside of your wrist and leave it on overnight to see if irritation does occur. If it does, then that herb is not for you.

Pregnant women should not use aromatherapy unless they have consulted a qualified aromatherapist.

Aromatherapy may, where appropriate, be combined pleasantly with Reflexology, where your body functions are said to be affected by massage of various parts of your feet. Sleep is associated with gentle massage of your toes and a few drops of olive oil with a relaxing scented addition does give great relaxation to adults. In babies there is no need for additional remedies. I have found that a gentle stroking of their toes between my thumb and fingers will pacify crotchety babies and often put them in the mood for sleep.

Bach Flower Remedies have also become a part of the herbalist's armamenterium.

In the 1930s Dr Edward Bach devised a system to classify people in seven main emotional groups. The emotions he listed were fear, uncertainty, disinterest in surroundings, self-centredness, oversensitivity to influences and ideas, despondency or despair and over-caringness for the welfare of others. Under these headings he listed a further thirty-eight negative states and formulated a plant- or flower-based remedy to treat each. These remedies he found in the Oxfordshire countryside where he lived, so their names are familiar to all of us who live in the Western hemisphere. There are no strengths available on the bottles of Bach Flower Remedies, but as the treatment recommended is to put only two drops in a glass of water or fruit juice it is likely that they are well diluted when taken. Two drops may also be dropped under the tongue or rubbed into the temples or wrists.

These remedies are not homeopathic. Unlike homeopathy, they treat the condition. They are not devised to mimic the illness. (Homeopathic theory will be described in the next chapter.) Suffice to say that Dr Bach's Remedies seem to fall more appropriately into the herbal section of this book. He suggests olive for tiredness and lack of energy; herbalists use the olive for insomnia. He suggests rock rose for terror; herbalists also feel that rose brings calm. He uses walnut for those who are oversensitive to change and outside influences; herbalists use walnut to encourage assertiveness. There is something very attractive about his idea that you get to know your failings, either by looking into yourself or by asking those near to you.

Then you find the remedy most suitable for your problem and keep it with you so that when it overwhelms you, you may use two drops to make yourself feel better.

In addition he brought out a combination of five Bach Flower Remedies: Rock Rose for terror; Impatiens for impatience; Clematis for dreaminess; Star of Bethlehem for the after-effects of shock; Cherry Plum for fear of the mind giving way, and he called this the Bach Rescue Remedy. It is to be used in times of upheaval. I met a conductor of a big orchestra who told me he had used it for years. I can think of few more stressful occupations. He certainly appeared very fit on it. My experience of these remedies is otherwise non-existent. They are not so much for sleep as to steady the personality defect that is causing insomnia. Thus you must decide first which emotional category you fall into and then which particular feeling is keeping you awake. Willow for resentment, elm for a feeling of being overwhelmed by responsibility, pine for self-reproach, sweet chestnut for mental anguish, larch for lack of confidence, the list may be found at any herbalist or pharmacy who stocks these remedies. A qualified herbalist would help you to find the right one. Again, seek expert help before you use them in pregnancy or if you are breast-feeding a baby.

Summary

> And still she slept an azure-lidded sleep,
> In blanched linen, smooth, and lavender'd,
>> *John Keats*

1. Taking herbs to make you sleep is like taking sleeping pills. If you need them, you should also try to find out why you are not sleeping and cure that.

2. Herbs act more slowly, so have to be taken for longer to gain effect. Herbs may have side effects just like stronger synthetic medicines.

3. Some herbal remedies for insomnia, such as almonds, olives, lettuce, barley water and porridge, are in our normal food supply and may be taken towards evening to encourage sleep.

4. Aromatherapy may encourage sleep without being addictive.

5. Reflexology may complement aromatherapy massage, or be used by itself.

6. Bach Flower Remedies are sold as a herbal treatment for emotional problems. Some may facilitate sleep.

7   Herbal remedies and teas not in our normal diet, Aromatherapy and Bach Flower Remedies should not be used by pregnant women or children without expert advice.

Case History

Jane used to drink coffee all day but last thing at night she had a cup of milky tea. She had no trouble getting to sleep until she stopped drinking so much coffee. After a few months of limiting her coffee intake to one cup in the morning, she began to find she went to bed and felt very wakeful. When she stopped her night-time tea she found she went to sleep without bother. She asked me for an explanation.

I felt that while she was taking a great deal of coffee her body got used to the constant state of stimulation and a cup of milky tea did not have much more effect even though she drank it at night. When she stopped the coffee her body, once it had lost its resistance to the coffee, began to react to the milder stimulation of her night-time tea. She did not really need anything to make her sleep but I suggested a warm milky drink or barley water if she fancied a warm drink last thing at night.

Chapter Six

Homeopathy

Christian Freidrich Samuel Hahneman (1775–1843) created the idea of Homeopathic medicine. Born in Dresden to a not very well off family, he none the less studied medicine and chemistry at Leipzig and Vienna and, as his experience in medical practice grew, so did his revulsion at the current treatments he was being taught to offer.

At the time, doctors had little understanding of the causation of disease, whether infectious, tumourous or from some hormonal imbalance. Treatment was by purgation, starvation and blood-letting.

Hahneman could see that calling in the doctor often lessened a patient's chances of recovery and certainly made the sufferer feel a great deal worse almost at once. He began to consult old texts and found a much more congenial approach to treatment in the writings of Paracelsus (1490–1541), an Italian physician. '*Similia similibus curantur*,' wrote Paracelsus: 'Similar things cure each other.'

Hahneman himself had noticed that quinine taken by a healthy person produced symptoms very like the malaria for which it was prescribed. He also noticed that few children with measles got whooping cough at the same time, although both diseases were rife in the community. He put forward the idea that, as both measles and whooping cough were illnesses with cough and fever, they excluded each other, protecting the body by their very presence. When a child recovered from one disease he might then catch the other. Hahneman said that this was because though similar, the diseases were not so very alike that the resistance acquired was complete. He had the experience of seeing a child with a chronic herpetic eruption completely cured of her problem by a dose of measles. In this case, he asserted, the acute illness with a rash, fever and perhaps cough had been so similar to the herpes that the resistance it stimulated had also affected the more chronic herpetic infection and driven it out too.

Convinced by these observations, Hahneman went on to write down his theory of medicine.

'The Physician's highest calling, his only calling, is to make sick people healthy, to heal as it is termed,' he wrote. He advised doctors not to waste time on fancy ideas and hypotheses which endeavoured to explain disease phenomena and causation.

Finding the cause of illness is the backbone of Western medicine. When Hahneman lived little was known and the equipment available was unable to isolate invading bacteria and viruses. Doctors were left to explain disease onset with theories of invasion by heat or cold or dampness. Hahneman spoke instead about a spirit-like force (*dynamis*) that in health reigns supreme within the body. 'Without this force,' he said, 'a body dies.'

Curing an illness was not just the elimination of all the symptoms and signs of the disease, said Hahneman. It was also necessary to remove the minor modifications of the vital force that had occurred. Only then could the physician be sure that the whole disease process was destroyed. He wanted his medicines to alter the way a person feels and functions. They must produce symptoms of the disease in the healthy and remove them from the sick. He went on to explain that in some cases a patient's symptoms might become more acute after treatment. This he called 'an aggravation' and was due purely to too powerful a dose. It would disappear spontaneously with withdrawal of the medication, when reassessment of the patient would then lead to the correct dose being offered. Hahneman felt that the curative value of his medicines depended on the symptoms they produced in the healthy being similar to those produced by disease, only stronger. In this way his medication would not just moderate the effect the disease was having on the vital force; it would extinguish and eradicate it. He had become strongly opposed to the current allopathic form of medicine being practised and denounced the three main treatments currently in vogue.

Blood letting, he said, merely led to further congestion; mercury had serious side effects and digitalis required higher and higher doses to remain effective.

At the time of writing he had a lot of right on his side. Conventional treatment by starvation and 'bleeding' must have removed what natural resistance a patient had to any affliction. His views, however, were not received with joy by his fellow physicians, who did their best to pour scorn on his ideas. Patients, on the other hand, found his theories pleasant and effective, so his practice flourished.

Hahneman took time with his patients. He took a history of the disease not only from the sufferer but from his friends and family, asking them if they had noticed any changes in his patient's nature or habits. It was necessary, said Hahneman, to study the patient's whole personality before prescribing, as the chosen medicine would depend not only on the complaint but his patient's temperament. Was he practical or dreamy; did he prefer hot or cold weather; was he an optimist or prone to depression? He would prescribe only one medicine at any one time. This is still current practice in Homeopathy, as Hahneman's treatment was called.

He insisted that his medicines should be tested by healthy people, both male and female, so their effects could be documented. At first Hahneman himself, his family and friends took on the duty of 'proving' his medicines, as the testing was called. They undertook to take no other medication, to eat only a simple nourishing diet without spices, greens, root vegetables, salad or soup herbs and to drink only water.

This 'Provers' Union' isolated twenty-six remedies and Hahneman started treatment with this original *materia medica*. It has since been enlarged to many hundreds of 'proved' medicines.

During these experiments he also found that as the solutions of his medicines became more dilute, their efficacy seemed to increase.

Making up homeopathic medicines is a very exact business. Soluble plant or animal extracts are dissolved in a mixture of alcohol and water. Insoluble minerals are triturated, ground so fine that they become soluble. These are allowed to stand for about three weeks before being strained off through a press. The resulting mother tincture is then diluted to different strengths. Even this process is done in a set way. The tinctures are diluted according to either the decimal scale (x) or the centesimal (c) and these signs are on all bottles to tell you what strength the contents are. In the decimal scale one drop of mother tincture is mixed with nine drops of an alcohol/water mixture and then a drop of that mixture is taken to be mixed with another nine drops of solute until the correct dilution is obtained. In the case of the centesimal scale one drop of mother tincture is mixed with ninety-nine drops of solute and a drop of that is taken to be dissolved in the next ninety-nine drops of solution. So to produce a 1c solution of Coffea, one drop of the mother tincture would be mixed with ninety-nine drops of alcohol/water mixture. For 2c you would take one drop of the 1c mixture and dilute it in another ninety-nine drops of solute. By the time you have got to 12c or 30x there may not be a single molecule of the original mother substance discenible in the mixture.

The method of mixing these solutions is also done in a special way. Hahneman called it succussion. He said it liberated the energy of the active substance. He shook the test tube of mixture vigorously and tapped it down on a book, making the solution jump. Once diluted to the correct amount, lactose tablets are swirled round in the mixture until they are fully impregnated with the solution. They are then placed in airtight dark glass bottles and, if stored away from direct sunlight, these tablets will last for some years.

Hahneman's theories were not new. The principal that like can cure like was put forward by Hippocrates in the fifth century BC and it may not have been new then. His theory became overruled by supporters of the Law of Contraries, by which men such as Galen tended to treat signs of disease with something that would prevent them. For instance, they would prescribe opium, which is very constipating, for diarrhoea. Paracelsus turned people again to the idea that like cures like. For diarrhoea he might have suggested castor oil which is a strong aperient. But again the Law of Contraries became more popular and through the middle ages herbs that controlled symptoms tended to be prescribed.

Hahneman's homeopathic theory is slightly different from Paracelsus's in that he teaches that the more dilute the medication the more potent. His medicines support the life force within us so that it may drive out invading forces that cause illness. The theory is perhaps closer to Eastern medicine, in which the balance of forces within our bodies is the important factor to maintain.

Western-trained doctors often feel uneasy about prescribing a medication in which they know there may not be any active substance present, but patients go by results and Dr Hahneman's medicines and way of treating patients became very popular, both in Germany and then through Europe, Britain and America. It fell into disuse when antibiotics were invented and Western medicine could suddenly cure some dangerous infections. Why rally your body's life force to resist pneumonia when a two-day course of antibiotic would completely cure it?

I believe its present resurgence in popularity follows the almost over-success of modern medicines. They are now so powerful and have such dangerous side effects that patients again wonder if they are not better off with a system of medicine that does not make them feel doubly ill because of the medication.

Although many allopathic trained doctors offer homeopathic medication, the attraction of this form of treatment is that it is cheap and may be bought over the counter at health food stores and chemists.

The rules are simple: take only one medication at a time. Do not handle the pills but put them on your tongue with a clean teaspoon and let them dissolve. Don't eat or drink for thirty minutes before taking homeopathic medicines and while under treatment eat a sensible nourishing diet. If you want to follow the diet of the Provers' Union, see it does not contain spices, greens, root vegetables, salads or soup herbs. Drink only water. Do not wear strong perfumes or use minty toothpaste while you are taking treatment either. The medication will then have its full effect.

Remember, the stronger effect should be obtained by using the more dilute 30x or over 12c. Because homeopathic medication works by increasing the body's own resistance as well as overcoming the invading force that is attacking your *dynamis*, it ceases to be needed when your vital force has returned to full health. The medication, therefore, should never become addictive. If it does, the taker is addicted to the form of treatment, not the medication itself. This is possible but is unlikely to be harmful where the medicine taken is so dilute that active substance is probably not present. However, if a homeopathic remedy for sleeplessness is not effective or seems to be needed continuously, it is wise to consult a qualified doctor, preferably trained in homeopathy, as insomnia may be a symptom of some more deep-seated malady.

To choose which remedy might help your insomnia you must first assess your own personality and the cause of your sleeplessness. If you find your mind overactive at night; if you find it difficult to relax and though you eventually get to sleep you toss and turn miserably before you do, then you might want to try coffea cruda (Coff)

This may be especially useful if your insomnia is due to the sudden emotion associated with good or bad news and you feel better lying down in the warmth and sucking ice cubes, and you feel worse if there is noise, cold air or strong smells about you and sleeping pills have not helped. Take coffea 30c one tablet an hour before you go to bed for ten nights. You may repeat the dose once if you wake and cannot get back to sleep.

If your insomnia is caused by stress or exhaustion and, though you fall asleep with no bother you also wake at three or four in the morning and cannot get back to sleep for a couple of hours, then you might try Nux vomica. To confirm the likelihood of this medication helping, you will probably also have nightmares and feel irritable and critical of others as well as having a pretty miserable outlook on life. Being left alone, warmth, and getting some sleep helps you and your best time of the day is the evening. Over-eating, over-indulgence in alcohol, cold wet weather and noise all make you feel worse. If this is you, try Nux vomica 30c. Take one tablet an hour before bed. Again you may repeat the dose once only if you wake and cannot get back to sleep.

If your insomnia is associated with fear and possibly caused by a shock or exposure to dry cold winds; if you feel restless, nervous, and have a fear of dying that induces nightmares and restless sleep, Aconite may suit you. In addition you will feel better in fresh air, worse in warm, tobacco smoke-filled rooms and worse in the evenings. You will not get any benefit from music. Try Aconite 30c taking one tablet an hour before bed. You may repeat the dose once only, if you wake and find it difficult to doze off again.

The insomnia that is accompanied by fear that you will never sleep again is different. Here you yawn but cannot sleep. You fear bedtime. Nightmares may affect your sleep and your moods change rapidly from over-loud laughter to crying. Emotional stress or grief are the usual cause of this sort of insomnia and you feel better after passing urine, eating or walking and worse after taking coffee or alcohol, if you are over warmly dressed, or in fresh cold air. For this sort of insomnia try Ignatia 30c, taking one tablet an hour before bed for ten nights and repeat the dose if you wake up and cannot get back to sleep.

Where depression is the main cause of your insomnia (especially in women at the menopause or premenstrually) and you feel weepy especially in the evening; if hot stuffy rooms and rich food make you feel worse while a cold drink or having a good cry or gentle exercise in the fresh air improves your mood, Pulsatilla 6c one tablet three times a day for two weeks may make you feel better.

Arsenicum album may be effective to treat the

insomnia that follows over-exertion, where you feel almost too tired to get to sleep. Try Arsen. alb. 30c one tablet twice a day for two weeks.

Most herbalists and pharmacies stock homeopathic remedies these days and are willing to advise you what to take. They are not expensive and in the highest dilutions, where no molecule of the active substance is present, they are probably safe for nursing mothers. In pregnancy it is sensible not to take any medication unless your doctor prescribes it. If these homeopathic remedies do not work after a week or so, you should consult your doctor about the problem. Even in great dilution an allergic reaction to these medications is possible so it is sensible to check with your doctor that you may try a homeopathic remedy before you take it.

Summary

Enjoy the honey-heavy dew of slumber.
William Shakespeare

1. Homeopathy is not Herbalism.

2. Homeopathy is based on the theory that 'like cures like' so medication gives the same symptoms as the disease it will cure if taken by healthy people.

The natural way to sound sleep

3. The more dilute the homeopathic remedy, the stronger is its potency. This is different from allopathic medicine, in which concentrated dosage is considered more effective.

4. Homeopathic remedies are readily available over the counter and because of their great dilution are generally free of side effects though 'aggravations' may occur where the patient's symptoms get suddenly worse. The medicine should then be stopped.

5. If the homeopathic treatment you think appropriate does not work or if your symptoms appear to get worse, you should consult your doctor.

6. If you are pregnant you should consult your doctor before you take any medication.

Case History

Mrs Smith was fifty-five and for five years had taken temazepam capsules to help her sleep. She started them after her menopause. At the time she had decided not to take hormone replacement, but had found her nights pretty miserable because of sweating attacks. She told me she had begged her doctor to give her something to get her to sleep and somehow she had just continued to ask for a repeat prescription.

She had read about temazepam being used as a drug of addiction and she was now unhappy about taking any more. Equally, she had tried coming off them before and had had some horrendous nights with wild dreams which had disturbed her very much.

I explained that when she stopped temazepam her rapid eye movement sleep would increase markedly for at least a month and she might experience bad dreams during this time.

She thought about it for a while and then asked if homeopathic medication could help this dreaming. We discussed her feelings and I came to realize that she was a very typical 'Ignatia' personality, sensitive and emotionally fragile. She had grieved when her menopause had, as she said, 'robbed her of youth' and had always hoped her periods would come back. She told me that if she didn't take her sleeping pills she found herself dreading bedtime. She felt tired, yawned all the time, but could not get to sleep.

I suggested she took Ignatia 30c, one tablet an hour before bed for the next two weeks.

She returned to tell me that for the first week there had been no improvement and she had scarcely slept. After that she had decided to tire herself and found she felt better for a good walk and in the second week her dreams had not been so upsetting. She did not feel that sense of 'knock out' with the Ignatia tablets that her temazepam had given her. She did feel much calmer and no longer dreaded bedtime. She decided she could now try to sleep without any pills. I suggested a hot milky drink before bed and she liked that idea. She is now off temazepam and sleeping normally.

Chapter Seven

The Chinese medical approach to insomnia

'We find that many people who offer us Chinese medical treatment are not qualified doctors,' said a man I met at a party.

'Are you unsatisfied with ordinary Western medicine?' I asked

'My wife feels that Western medicine cures illness but Chinese medicine will prevent it arising.'

He had a point.

Chinese medicine is based on the *Nei Jing*, the bible of Chinese medicine, just as Western medicine is described in huge tomes such as *The Oxford Textbook of Medicine*.

The difference is that Western text books are rewritten every few years, as doctors learn new causations and cures of disease, while the *Nei Jing* is added to and modified but the basic principles hold as good today as they did about 200 BC when it was first written.

Chinese doctors are interested in maintaining each person in a harmonious state, as a house looks its best if its architecture is balanced within itself and in accord with its environment. They are not interested in isolating a particular invading virus and providing specific medicine to destroy it, allowing the body to then recover its health.

They will try rather to repair the imbalance visible in their patient and in that way allow his own returning strength to drive out an invading influence.

As a doctor, trained in Western medicine, I found it hard to have confidence in this approach. Yet as I read more and more, I could see that this different way of thinking could have many advantages. As so often in medicine the middle way is again being proved the correct one. It is horses for courses and there are many afflictions where the Chinese approach is being shown to be as or more effective than the Western.

Which of you has not heard of a friend whose chronic pain has been relieved by acupuncture when physiotherapy has failed, or whose eczema has been ameliorated by herbs from a Chinese doctor when Western emollients and cortisone creams have proved ineffective?

The Chinese use both herbs and acupuncture (or moxibustion) to restore body equanimity and the correct use of these is important and requires training.

Both treatments are powerful and though a 'blockbuster' approach by an amateur may have a satisfactory outcome, this is not being treated in a Chinese medical way. In Western medicine the equivalent to this approach would be for an untrained person to hand out one of the proton pump inhibitors to anyone with indigestion or stomach discomfort. Because they are very effective most people would notice an improvement in their symptoms and think they were cured. However, those whose pain was due to an early cancer or a resistant ulcer would just be covering up their symptoms and the disease process would continue unabated until correct diagnosis and full treatment got to the root of the problem. It might by then be too late to save that patient. However the person who was handing out the proton pump inhibitors would have made a great name for himself as a medicine man because there are many more simple cases of indigestion than there are more serious conditions and these drugs have a wide and powerful effect.

Do-it-yourself acupuncture and treatment with herbs whose side effects you have no knowledge of is dangerous. This chapter is not offering you that sort of expertise. I will explain the way Chinese doctors approach the diagnosis

and treatment of their patients so that you may
make up your mind whether this approach is for
you. Medical students in the Western world
have a long training and it is the same for
practitioners of Chinese medicine.

Traditional Chinese medicine – as Western –
is both an art and a science. The theory is based
on everything being in balance with its equal
and opposite. This is the Yin/Yang theory. Each
person is like a little world and in health the
forces within him or her are in comfortable
balance and in tune with the surroundings to
give a strong, content individual. Should either
your Yin or Yang become too powerful or
dwindle away, your body forces become unbalanced, your organs don't work normally and
you are left open to invasion by destructive
influences. Maintaining this inner balance is
therefore of constant importance and any devia-
tion requires instant treatment – the very
essence of Western holistic preventative medicine. The Yin/Yang theory is not hard to accept.
You all know that, as well as food, sleep and
exercise, happiness, sadness, ambition and disinterest also have an effect on physical growth
and repair and mental health. The Chinese have
rationalized these triggering events into the Yin
element, representing the sheltered, shadowy
side of a hill and the Yang, the sunny, exposed
side. So Yin elements in life are cold, dark,

inferiority and decrease, and are associated with the interior of your body; Yang aspects are heat, excitement, activity and light and are associated with your skin.

Following this concept it is possible to separate a Yin dominated problem from a Yang though where one element is dominant the cause may be due to weakness of the other element rather than an absolute increase in its strength.

The Yin/Yang theory extends to cover your whole world. Night is Yin: day is Yang. Depression is Yin: euphoria is Yang. You feel cold and

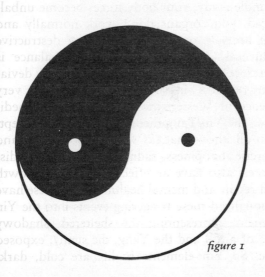

figure 1

sad when your Yin is in ascendance, hot and agitated when your Yang is overpowerful. When they are in balance, you feel comfortable happy and active.

The Taoist picture of Yin and Yang in balance shows a static picture (see fig. 1).

The Chinese realize this is a figure that is constantly in movement with equal and opposites always finding a balance. The little circles of Yin/Yang within their opposite colours are to remind you that within the major concept of Yin and Yang there can also be Yin elements of Yang and Yang elements of Yin, which are finding their own equilibrium within the whole organism. If this is opaque, remember your overwhelming joy when you heard that you had passed an exam or got a job. This is Yang but within it is the Yin feeling of self-satisfaction at the solid work you put in to get this result. However if you were disappointed by failing to achieve a result you would be in a Yin state but that self same feeling of self-satisfaction at having done your best would now appear uplifting and Yang. Either way as time passes your wilder feelings moderate and as a concentrated solution disperses within a more dilute one, the Yin and Yang of your moods and emotions tend naturally to even out to restore your body's balance.

While the Yin/Yang theory encompasses

everything around you, the Chinese believe that you also have specific principles governing your body that act to keep it in harmony.

Qi is your body's power source. It is a concept, not something you can see or touch.

Qi is the force responsible for keeping your bodies sound and in healthy normal growth. It motivates talk, thought, activity and development. In health it is always in movement, penetrating every part of you, going up and down, entering and leaving.

Qi resists invasion of your body by pernicious influences and masterminds the production of blood, urine and sweat from the digestion and reformulation of your food. It maintains your body temperature and controls the working of all your organs. Think of Qi as the conductor of your body's orchestra.

Chinese doctors have five main categories of Qi. Organ Qi is specialized to the main organs and controls their position and action. Nutritive Qi flows with the blood to help digestion of food to form blood elements. Protective Qi combats the attack of pernicious influences ever ready to invade the body and Ancestral Qi regulates heartbeat and respiration. Channel Qi flows in pathways associated with organs called channels or meridians. This concept is the basis for acupuncture treatment.

These channels or meridians are an invisible

network that carry the concept Qi throughout the body so that it can do its work.

There are twelve main channels connected with the main organs but many other minor channels have been mapped out.

Within these the Qi runs smoothly in health. When disharmony occurs the Qi may not be able to perform its duties. If it lies stagnant in its channels or flows in the wrong direction bodily malfunctions result.

Chinese doctors accept the idea of blood flow through the body but their map of its circulation is different to that in Western texts and they place more importance on the relationship of blood with the major organs such as the heart, liver and spleen. The Chinese also talk about Jing, the building blocks of organic life.

Prenatal Jing is inherited and determines how you will grow. You get your postnatal Jing from the food you eat and it reinforces the power of your prenatal Jing.

Jing controls your body's form through childhood growth spurts, strong young adulthood into withered old age. It is, in a sense, the physical manifestation of Qi. A Chinese patient of mine was telling me about her son, 'His Jing is strong now that he is a man,' she said. 'He was such a weakly baby.'

Shen is your essential personality and spirit. It is what a doctor sees first when you visit him, when he notices whether your eyes are bright and interested and your walk powerful or if you drag into the room with downcast face.

When general disharmony of Yin and Yang occurs your body's defences are weakened and pernicious influences may invade. These influences are wind, cold, fire and heat, dampness, dryness and summer heat. They may attack from inside or outside, making you feel unwell enough to call in the doctor. He will endeavour to right the imbalance in your body that has allowed invasion so that your own system will be strong enough to counter the pernicious influence.

This has similarities with the Western holistic treatment approach, and before you turn your nose up about pernicious influences you should remember that your own Western medical system was based on Humours.

Joy, anger, grief and fear are emotions that the *Nei Jing* quotes as precipitating disharmony. Western medical experts would entirely agree. For instance, doctors in the West are well aware that long term grief, unresolved, may lead to depressive illness, bowel disorders and chronic pain. Treatment of these conditions is never successful unless the underlying grief reaction is ameliorated.

How do Chinese doctors go about their diagnosis?

They go through four stages: looking, listening and smelling, asking, and touching.

Facial colour, physical shape, skin condition and most important, the state of the tongue are all noted.

Under listening and smelling the doctor will assess the patient's way of speaking, time his respiration and note any cough or unusual sound. Rapid breathing, forceful speech and the rank smell of adrenalin-caused sweat suggests a Yang overaction; slow speech and depressed effect with a sour smell about the body presage Yin disharmony.

The doctor will go on to take a history much like his Western colleague. He is interested in past history and family history as well as the current malaise.

He will then examine his patient by touching various acupuncture points to assess the skin condition and he will take his patient's pulse at the wrist.

Taking the patient's pulse and examining his tongue are the most important parts of the examination. These are diagnostic skills that doctors in Western medicine have largely lost relying instead on laboratory tests to tell them what is wrong with a patient.

It is horses for courses. In the vast continent of China there are not facilities available for Western-type diagnoses. Observation and examination of a patient become of paramount importance, just as they were in the West a century ago. Medicine is still both art and science. In the West doctors should not forget this, nor rely totally on machinery to make their decisions for your treatment.

At the end of the examination the Chinese physician feels he has found the reason for his patient's disharmony and sets about treating it with acupuncture or moxibustion and herbs.

Acupuncture is the insertion of fine needles into points along the channels or meridians that have been mapped out by trial and error over hundreds of years. Moxibustion is the same technique using heat applications at acupuncture points. Usually the herb burned is mugwort (*artemesia vulgaris*) and the patient feels a pleasant warmth at the site. These two treatments are looked on as Yang as they work from the outside in. Herbs taken internally are Yin. Both work, not to cure the complaint, but to rebalance your body's Yin/Yang status so that your complaint disappears. Chinese physicians feel that insomnia is most often due to deficient Heart Blood or deficient Heart Yin. Both cause disturbed sleep and wild dreams.

If your problem is deficient Heart Blood you are likely to have a weak pulse and pale tongue and that uneasy feeling that you have forgotten to do something you should have. This brings difficulty in getting to sleep but once you get over, your sleep is undisturbed. It may be associated with a deficient Spleen Qi which has much the same symptoms but often includes a poor appetite. Anxiety may cause this sort of sleep loss. Patients with a deficient Heart Yin have all the signs of a dominant Yang, a reddish tongue, warm hands, a rapid pulse and palpitations. Their problem is not only going to sleep but remaining asleep because their weak Yin has allowed the pernicious influence, heat, to enter and disturb their Shen or spirit. Deficient Kidney Yin with its additional symptoms of irritability, backache, sweating and ringing in the ears may be associated with deficient Heart Yin. Hormonal imbalances such as an overactive thyroid or menopausal flushings might give these symptoms.

In addition these disharmonies may also be connected to other organs which is why so many different acupuncture points are offered to treat insomnia in different alternative medicine books.

Insomnia with early morning waking and an everpresent feeling of fear may sound like depression to us but would probably be diagnosed as either deficient Heart Qi or deficient Gall Bladder Qi.

You all know the insomnia that is associated

with abdominal discomfort, a feeling of bloat-
ing and a greasy feeling in the mouth. It may
follow a heavy meal last thing at night but if it
becomes chronic Western doctors consider irritable bowel syndrome with its irregular stool
and belching. The Chinese doctor talks of an
unharmonized stomach.

The insomnia that occurs when you lie angry
and railing against what the world has done to
you is associated with disharmony of the Liver
or Gallbladder say the Chinese. Sleep is impossible. Your pulse bounds, your head aches and
you have a bitter taste in your mouth.

These are all recognizable forms of insomnia.
The terminology is different and the diagnosis
highly specific because in China the simple
sleeping pill to override symptoms is not an
option. Treatment must bring the whole person
back to a comfortable equilibrium, mental and
physical. Acupuncture and herbal medicines, the
mainstay of Chinese medical treatment, would
be their prescription.

If you feel that you would like your insomnia
investigated and treated within the discipline of
Chinese medicine it is essential to attend a
qualified practitioner just as you would if you
were seeking a Western-trained doctor.

'Do-it-yourself' acupuncture is not to be
recommended. There is a risk of infection where
the needles enter the skin. However, acupressure

over the same points with, say, a cotton bud or the tip of a finger, gently applied, so as not to cause a bruise, may give much the same result.

Can you give yourself acupressure?

Yes. But like an untrained person trying to perform manipulation you might not get either the diagnosis or the manoeuvre right. It would be wiser to start with a qualified physician's opinion and treatment and then, if he allows, reinforce his treatment by repeating it.

It is possible to apply acupressure to oneself. You may use a cotton bud or your finger or thumb end.

Cut your nails short on the finger you are going to use. As the channels or meridians run equally on both sides of your body you may have to use a finger or thumb from each hand to reach the acupressure points comfortably. Apply the top of the finger, not the pulp. Feel round for the area of greatest sensitivity at the given points. You press in at right angles to the skin unless otherwise directed and offer counterclockwise rotation at the point. The skin should move under your finger pressure. If possible do not bruise the tissue. Acupressure should not be done every day. The tissue would become damaged. Once is enough to clear the channel you think is blocked. A second time might reblock it. Allow at least a week between treatments at any one point. Acupressure should

USEFUL ACUPUNCTURE POINTS

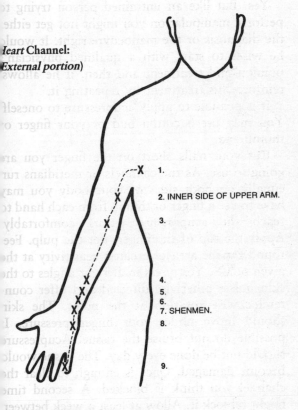

Heart Channel:
(External portion)

1.

2. INNER SIDE OF UPPER ARM.

3.

4.
5.
6.
7. SHENMEN.
8.

9.

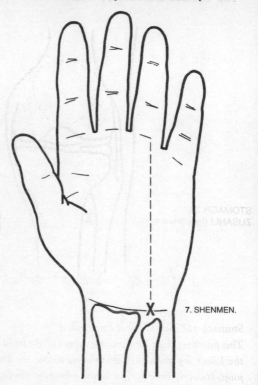

7. SHENMEN.

Heart 7: Shenmen (*gate of the spirit*)

This point is found on the transverse crease on the 'little finger' side of the wrist. It lies almost in line with the base of your ring finger when you hold your hand out flat with the palm up.

It is used to treat insomnia, pain in the upper abdomen and chest, hysteria, amnesia, and palpitations.

132

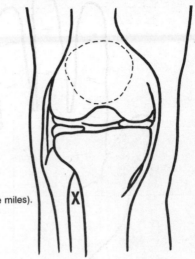

STOMACH 36.
ZUSANLI (foot three miles).

Stomach 36: Zusanli (*foot three miles*)

This point is found on the outer aspect of the front of the lower leg about 1.5 centimetres below the knee joint. It overlies the dip just below where the tibia and fibula join at the top of the lower leg.

This is an often used acupuncture point, not only for insomnia but also for hypertension, aching legs, gastric pain and dizziness. It has health promoting properties and relieves nervous tension and stress.

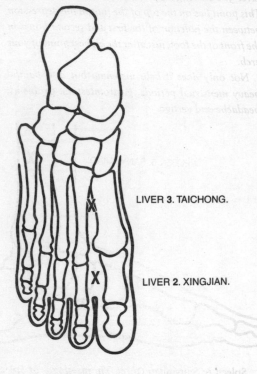

LIVER 3. TAICHONG.

LIVER 2. XINGJIAN.

Liver 2: Xingjian
This point lies on the web between the first and second toes and helps insomnia and hypertension.

Liver 3: Taichong (*imperial communications centre*)
This point lies on the top of the foot in the depression between the junction of the first and second bones in the front of the foot, just after the highest point of your arch.

Not only does it help insomnia but also painful heavy menstrual periods, gastrointestinal problems, headache and vertigo.

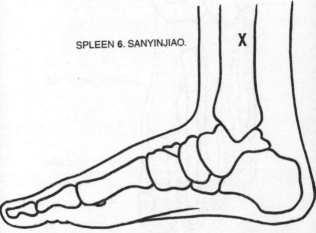

SPLEEN 6. SANYINJIAO.   X

Spleen 6: Sanyinjiao (*three Yin meeting – of Spleen, Liver and Kidney Channels*)
This point should not be compressed or needled or heated in any pregnant woman.

It lies on the inner side of the lower leg about two inches above the most prominent part of the inner ankle bone and acts to relieve abdominal distension (hence not to be used during pregnancy) and to relieve insomnia.

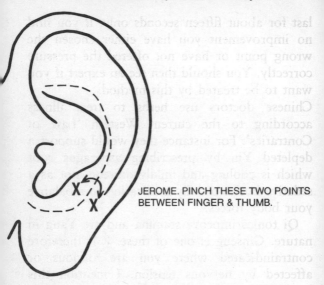

JEROME. PINCH THESE TWO POINTS
BETWEEN FINGER & THUMB.

Jerome: (*pinch these two points between finger &
thumb*)
*Auricular acupuncture and acupressure have recently
become fashionable. The Chinese believe that the
whole body can be represented, curled up in foetal
position, within the ear. This means that pain or
trouble within the body may be relieved by pressure or
needling at certain points on the ear. These are
necessarily very close to each other so great experience
is needed to get it right but helpful points to ameliorate
insomnia such as 'Jerome' and others have been
mapped out. Some lie just on the skull behind the
lower root of the ear and some lie in the auricle as
shown above. It is not wise to put pressure on these
sensitive skull areas but a gentle massage of the back of
the head behind the ears relieves stress and ameliorates
tension headache.*

last for about fifteen seconds only. If you find no improvement you have either chosen the wrong point or have not offered the pressure correctly. You should then see an expert if you want to be treated by this method.

Chinese doctors use herbs to treat illness according to the current Western 'Law of Contraries'. For instance they would support a depleted Yin by prescribing asparagus root which is cooling and mildly diuretic, not as a sedative but as a daily medication to rebalance your body forces.

Qi tonics improve stamina and are Yang in nature. Ginseng is one of these. It is therefore contraindicated where you are anxious or affected by nervous tension. I mention this because so many people think of Ginseng as a panacea and by taking it for insomnia could be making their condition worse.

Sleeplessness is generally treated with Xue tonics which are more in line with the condensing and sinking herbs of modern herbal medicine. Chinese angelica (dang gui) is one of these. It relaxes the stress of work or trauma and is a peripheral vasodilator so has a blood pressure lowering action. Rehmannia (Chinese foxglove) is another Xue remedy, especially for deficient Kidney Yin. It is said to cool 'the heat in the heart' which presents as insomnia, irritability, a flushed face and a tendency to mouth ulcers.

Peony root and mulberries are other cooling Xue remedies. Chinese herbs are prescribed not for the single symptom of sleeplessness and a Chinese physician will put together a herbal mixture that has an overall effect to achieve rebalance between your Yin and Yang. My strong advice to any reader who wants to try Chinese medical treatment is to turn first to a fully trained practitioner. You can find one in your area by contacting The Council for Complementary and Alternative Medicine, whose present address is Suite D, Park House, 206–208 Latimer Road, London W10 6RE. Taking remedies of whose contents and actions you have no real knowledge is not sensible. Seek expert advice.

Summary

> I haven't been to sleep for over a year. That's why I go to bed early. One needs more rest if one doesn't sleep.
>
> *Evelyn Waugh*

1. Illness is caused by disharmony in your body. A Chinese physician will seek to rebalance your Yin and Yang.

2. To do this he may offer you herbal treatment, perhaps accompanied by acupuncture or moxibustion.

3. It is unwise to attempt to cure yourself with prepacked Chinese herb preparations without expert medical advice.

4. Acupuncture and moxibustion also require an expert but acupressure may be attempted gently on yourself using a cotton bud or thumb pressure over appropriate acupuncture points.

5. Gentle massage over acupuncture points that are associated with relief of sleeplessness may give a feeling of comfort and drowsiness and this massage may be combined with aromatherapy to encourage sleep. This is easier and safer for an untrained person to do. Better to leave acupressure to the experts.

Chapter Eight

Sleep and Ayurvedic medicine

Ayurvedic medicine has its origins in Hinduism and stems from the Indian subcontinent. Brahma, the first God of the trinity whose other members are Vishnu and Shiva, has four faces representing the four Vedas, the chief Hindu scriptures. The sacrificial spoon, beads and manuscript that he holds in his hands show him to be God of piety and wisdom. He may be recognized as a bearded, four-faced, four-armed old man sitting on a lotus supported by a swan. His wife, Sarasvati, is goddess of learning.

Brahma is the grandfather of gods and men, the creator god, who is said to have handed down the theory of Ayurvedic medicine to other gods and eventually to Atri, a worthy man, who in turn passed his knowledge to his son Bhagawan Panarvasu Atreya.

Atreya lived about 700 BC; with the help o

his disciples he wrote down his father's teachings. A century later it was edited, added to and refined by a physician called Caraka, almost certainly assisted by a committee of other experts. This edition was named the *Caraka Samhita*. A century after that a physician, Drdhabala, reconstructed the writings to give an amazingly modern look. He separated the text into eight sections: Fundamentals, Diagnosis, Specific features, Human body, Fatal signs, Treatment, Medicaments and Drugs, and Successful Management.

In the huge land mass of the Indian subcontinent, where poverty or wealth and health or illness were closely related to good or bad harvests and climatic conditions, the creator god soon became less interesting. Vishnu, the Preserver, who fought the dragon of drought and saved mankind in ten separate incarnations, gained popularity. So did Siva, the destroyer god, lord of spirits, protector of cattle, god of letters and music and dancing.

Siva's wife, Kali Durga, also gained many devotees intent on avoiding her ministrations with prayer and offerings. She is the dark mother, goddess of death and destruction, whose black, four-armed statue with its red palms, eyes and tongue and blood-stained breasts and matted hair is seen very frequently in India. She wears a necklace of skulls, earrings of corpses and a girdle of snakes. In eastern India around Calcutta, in Nepal and in Rajasthan, the Kalipuja on the darkest night of November is a scene of terror and placation when cattle and fowl are sacrificed to this rapacious queen.

Having been created, Brahma has given us the best he can. For most people it then becomes more important to stay alive and to prosper at work than to dwell on re-creation. The devotees of Brahma the creator dwindled as those of Vishnu and Shiva grew. However his teachings about medicine remained, were handed down and refined and still exist under the same headings set up so many ages ago.

Eight specialities were described: Internal Medicine, Surgery, Diseases of the head and neck, Children's and Women's problems, Toxicology, Invading spirits (and micro-organisms), Promotion of health by preventive care and Aphrodisiacs. Remembering that this system was introduced to deal with a very poor population in a country with violent temperature swings throughout the year coupled with catastrophic droughts and floods, where life expectancy was low and infectious disease rife rapid and frequently fatal, I am amazed how close to modern medical treatment these ancient texts are.

They postulate a healthy balance of mind

inner self and body as protective against illness. Nothing should be carried to excess. Their theme is that longevity and health depend on a regular, moderate lifestyle. The aims in life they seek to encourage are a desire for life, the pursuit of wealth and self-preparation for rein-carnation into the afterworld.

This apparent dichotomy with Christianity, where a rich man has as much chance of achieving Heaven as a camel getting through an eye of a needle, becomes less sharp when we realize that the pursuit of wealth is merely encouragement to work hard all one's life. It is governed by the stricture to prepare for one's next life, where reincarnation to a better state is totally dependent on behaviour in this world, so that wealth well used for general benefit works positively for hope of a better reincarnation. Given this qualification, there is a lot to be said for working with reward in prospect. We have proved the association of being jobless with ill health, and the malaise that often follows sudden retirement is well documented.

At the same time Ayurvedic medical writing advises against over-indulgence in anything, from work to thinking. The theory behind this accepts that the natural forces that maintain the world, such as the power that shakes the trees, makes the tops of mountains move and keeps bodily functions going, are always prepared to invade in force and destabilize the body. They must be kept out or allowed in only in the correct amounts. Keeping a healthy balance of sleep, eating and activity maintains health and prevents them overwhelming the constitution.

The forces that may overwhelm the body physically, Vata (wind or air), Pitta (bile or fire) and Kapha (phlegm or water) can be controlled and driven back by medication; those forces that attack the mind may be subdued by concentration.

Ayurvedic medicine uses drugs, topical treatments, massage and baths to treat diseases. The theory of treatment is not so much to attack the invading force as to strengthen the body's reserve so that it may return to its normal vigour and drive out the invading force or subdue its activity to what is normal and healthy.

Medicaments are many and varied. Animal, mineral and vegetable products are all listed. Those of animal origin range from honey, milk, bile, muscle and fat to urine, faeces, skin and hoof. These are both drunk and used topically. Sheep or goat urine is a very commonly prescribed draught, as is yoghurt and honey. Minerals include gold, silica, gem stones, ochre and galena. Vegetable medications may be made from fruit, seeds, leaves, bark, roots, tubers or latex. They may be swallowed raw, cooked or taken as the ash of the burned product. All these are also used topically.

The Ayurvedic pharmacopeoa is enormous, built and recorded through the ages by trial and error to suit the health problems of this particular area. The usual reason for such a huge choice is that none are particularly effective, but in this case it may be that the fauna and flora vary so markedly from area to area that different treatments have had to be offered in different parts of the country. There are about 600 listed evacuants alone, and as many for boils and fevers. Another reason for variety may lie in the caste system. This has been in place for over 3,000 years, dividing the population into strict groups with their own taboos and behaviour. Brahmins, the superior caste, are usually strongly vegetarian, and so their medication would have to be tailored with this in mind.

Sleep comes way down the list of importance in Ayurvedic medicine. This is not to say that its importance is minimized. Rather, that an Ayurvedic physician is consulted more often by patients with the catastrophic diseases common to tropical countries than by a simple insomniac. In addition, where daytime sleeping is common, people do not notice the loss of good night-time sleep. However, the Ayurvedic text is aware that sleep supports and protects and that over-indulgence in thought, or overwork, or a disease occurring at night, can interfere with this process. The text suggests that insomnia caused by overwork and physical illness must be cured by medication: sleeplessness due to over-indulgence in thought is considered a sin and must be controlled by mental concentration.

Ayurvedic medicine has four regulations for things and people involved in a disease process that are as true now as they were then. The physician must know his medical theory, have extensive experience, be dexterous and clean. The patient must have a good memory for the care he has received, must be obedient to his physician, fearless and provide all the information he has about his illness. His attendant must know how to look after a sick person, be dexterous, loyal and clean. The drugs offered must be plentifully available, effective, come in various pharmaceutical forms and be reproducible to a standard composition. Doctor or patient could not ask for more today.

Physicians were aware of the ingredients that lead to a sound sleep. The Ayurvedic text speaks of ensuring mental ease, a comfortable room and a well-covered bed. It suggests sleep can be helped by pleasant sounds, smells and gentle massage. Meat soup from domestic, marshy or aquatic animals is recommended, as is rice and curd, wine, milk and fat.

Purgation, emesis, fear, anxiety, anger, exercise, smoking, blood letting, fasting and an uncomfortable bed are listed as factors preventing good sleep. Old age, illness and overwork are also mentioned. Our own sleep hygiene leaflets are very similar.

Ayurvedic medicine distinguishes eight types of people more at risk of medical problems: the over-tall or short; the over-hairy or hairless; the over-dark or fair; and the over-fat or thin.

Again, there is a basis of truth in most of these groups being at special risk. The text associates poor sleep with being too fat or thin and we know that when dieting, sleep is interfered with. Dependent on good sleep, says the Veda, is happiness, strength, potency, intelligence, good health and longevity. Modern medicine would agree.

In the context of the climate it was written in, the text suggests very sensibly that sleeping during the day in summer is to be recommended and those to whom the siesta is a normal habit should continue with it all year.

Following most of these treatments would not take us far from Western medical recommendation. The medicaments, however, are not easily available and Ayurvedic trained doctors are scarce in the Western hemisphere. None the less, achieving a balance in your diet and in your daily lifestyle is a sensible way to maintain your health and stabilize your sleep pattern.

Ayurvedic doctors think that certain foods have antagonistic properties. These are often very different from combinations the West indulges in. Ayurvedic medical law suggests that fish and milk should not go together. Pigeon flesh and mustard oil go well together but should not be mixed with honey and milk, nor should sour liquids be mixed with milk. They even proscribe hot water and honey; this with whisky and lemon juice is a time-honoured toddy in Scotland and not taking honey and hot water would not appeal to a lot of Scots.

Depression as a cause of insomnia was well known. Ayurvedic text speaks of curing this sort of mental illness by religious readings and purposeful words. In the West you would call this counting your blessings and filling your mind with other people's words to block your own thoughts.

If this did not work, the doctor would go on to frighten his patient either by standing him in front of charging elephants, or telling him that the King had ordered his execution, or covering him in mustard oil and leaving him in the sun. In all these cases, when the patient found that these terrible things were not to be, or that his blistering skin was to be cured, his relief chased his depression away. In the West this is not dissimilar to aversion therapy.

Although you cannot readily make use of these remedies, the theory behind them backs a moderate life as offering a normal peaceful sleep and a good day. The dietary advice is sound and their use of massage and scent is possibly the origin of aromatherapy.

Summary

How do people go to sleep? I'm afraid I've lost the knack. I might try busting myself smartly over the temple with the nightlight. I might repeat to myself, slowly and soothingly, a list of quotations beautiful from minds profound; if I can remember any of the damn things.

Dorothy Parker

1. The Ayurvedic medical discipline dates from at least 700 BC.

2. It seeks to maintain a balance within your body between the forces within and all around you.

3. Its pharmacopoea is enormous, which may mean that because of the huge variation of plants and animals and minerals throughout the

Indian subcontinent different combinations had to be found for each area, or that none of them were very effective.

4. The dietary and sleep hygiene suggestions are very similar to those offered in Western medical practice.

5. If you want to be treated by a doctor skilled in Ayurvedic medicine you should approach the Council for Complementary and Alternative Medicine or an equivalent body in whichever country you are, for the name of a qualified practitioner.

Chapter Nine

A Tibetan
medical outlook

Buddha is said to have abandoned his sheltered princely life in quest of an answer to the origin of suffering when he saw a gnarled old man, a sick person and a funeral procession and became aware of the sorrows of life. In his Enlightenment he offered all men the 'Four Sublime Truths'. These, like a medical examination, go on from isolation of the cause to its eradication. He offered an 'Eight-fold Path', with concrete suggestions on how this might be achieved. His monks ministered to the community, gradually building these teachings into a medical discipline. Their teachings came to be written down as the *Tantra of Secret Instructions on the Eight Branches, the Essence of the Elixir of Immortality*, more usually referred to as the *Four Tantras*.

This treatise, which may have started as early as 889 AD, was edited by the regent Sangye

Gyamtso in about 1688 and illustrated with paintings to become an authoritative medical text called the *Blue Beryl*. Following the *Four Tantras*, it is divided up into the 'Root Tantra', which is a synopsis of medical teaching; the 'Exegetical Tantra', which deals with bodily structure and function; the 'Instructional Tantra', which offers treatment methods and medicines; and the 'Subsequent Tantra', which instructs the physician in how to diagnose and treat various illnesses. Together, the *Blue Beryl* and the *Four Tantras* form the origin of modern Tibetan medicine. They provide a rational and ordered discipline to live by, taking in not only the treatment of disease but explaining natural phenomena, organic pathology, psychology and the world around us within a systemized framework. The theory may not be totally in tune with Western teaching, but it is rational, respectable and impressive. Many of the teachings about sleep and dreaming, written in the seventeenth century if not before, are only now being appreciated and included in Western psychology books.

Buddhists feel that your body, feelings, perceptions, impulses and consciousness come together in a constantly changing mix to make you what you are. Your consciousness is the central part of your being and it is this that transmigrates from one existence to the next after death. Tibetans go on to believe that all substances have their origin in some mixture of five elements, earth, fire, water, air and space. These five elements are appreciated by one of your five senses and have a special affinity with that sense.

The 'Root Tantra' explains these principles and the humoural basis for illness. It also lays out four methods of treatment, by diet, by conduct, by medication and by external therapy. Of these, unless you are a qualified physician, only diet and conduct come into the do-it-yourself category. Yet they may be sufficient to help you to get over insomnia without further medication, so it is worth considering following their precepts.

In Tibetan medical thought our bodies are governed by three constitutional forces.

Air (*rLung*) maintains the subtle flow of vital energy in the body. It governs your emotional and spiritual make-up and imbalance of this energy within your body leads to psychological problems. People in whom this force is predominant are usually bluish complexioned, short, thin, extrovert characters, sexually active and pugnacious. They suffer from insomnia and the 'Exegetical Tantra' likens them to foxes, crows and vultures and says that they will never become wealthy and tend to live short lives.

Their food preferences are for sweet, sour and bitter foods.

Bile (*rKrispa*) promotes digestion and balances the body temperature to maintain it at the right heat. Bile provides the driving force behind your ambitions. Imbalance causes bowel and body heat disturbance. People who are governed predominantly by this force are sharp minded, proud and prone to hatred with yellowish skin and hair. They sweat a lot and have a tendency to feel hungry and thirsty all the time, longing for sweet, bitter and astringent foods. They resemble tigers and yaks and monkeys, says the 'Tantra', and live normal lives without extreme wealth.

Phlegm (*bekan*), controller of the elements of earth and water in the body, balances body fluids. It regulates the flow of mucus in your body and controls your joint fluids and so their flexibility. It also monitors your immune system to keep it in good working order to repel invasion from outside organisms. Imbalance of this humour leads to water retention, digestive problems and arthritis. The Tantra suggests that people dominated by phlegm are plump, fair complexioned, kind individuals. They are hard to ruffle, able to endure discomfort and may become wealthy and live long lives. They tend to sleep a great deal and are associated with lions and elephants and herd leaders.

Taking these three constitutional types as well as those types where there is a mixture of these constitutions with one dominant as well as one where there is parity, Tibetan medicine recognizes eight constitutions whose temperament is mainly that of the dominant force. These forces are kept in proportion within your body by seven sustaining processes which begin with the essence from your nutrients, which become blood products, which in turn form muscle tissue which begets bone. From bone comes marrow which forms regenerative fluid.

In examining patients Tibetan doctors place great importance on checking the urine. Together with an examination of the pulse, and an examination of the tongue, urinalysis enables the doctor to assess whether his patient is too hot or too cold and to prescribe 'hot' herbs or 'cold' herbs to rectify his body state.

Tibetan medicines are made from minerals and herbs. They are usually in pill form and are taken by crushing the pill and swallowing it in a little hot water. Turquoise, pearls, gold, primula, orchid and gentian are but a few of the substances used. These are not for do-it-yourself medicators. The herbs chosen have six primary tastes, eight potencies, seventeen qualities and three post-digestive effects. Their use should be left to doctors holding a qualification from the Tibetan Medical and Astrological Institute in

Dharamsala, India and if you visit a Tibetan doctor it is sensible to ask to see his or her qualification diploma. Alternatively, the Office of Tibet in London may offer advice.

Tibetans feel insomnia is caused by an imbalance of body processes. Most commonly the *rLung* is at fault. It may be that you go on to require medication but before you do you should make sure that your food intake, the basis of all body balance, is correct.

Tibetan medical texts suggest that all food comes from the five elements, fire, earth, water, air and space.

Water and earth make sweet foods such as sugar, meat, milk, grains and fruit. These foods tend to form the bulk of your diet and are considered by Tibetans, as well as in the West, to be the most nutritious of your daily intake. Tibetans say that these 'sweet' foods increase your energy and give you the power to do your daily work without feeling tired. They improve your skin and complexion, giving you the glowing look of health and they strengthen your eyesight. Taken in the right amount they promote relaxation, reduce anxiety, help soothe sore throats and stop coughs.

Over-indulge in these 'sweet' foods at your peril. Too much of them and you may suffer from any of the diseases associated with obesity such as heart problems, kidney and liver disorders, and arthritis. You may get diabetes, your thyroid gland may disfunction so that you get a goitre, you may even get swollen glands. Tooth decay, chronic sinusitis and skin problems are also the sequaelae of eating too much of this taste group.

Fire and earth make sour tastes. These scour the body channels and clear them. They aid digestion, and reduce mucus in the throat and lung passages as well as in the bowel. Sour tastes are yoghurt, cheese, and oranges and lemons. Take too much of these sour-tasting foods and Tibetans say you may get irritable skin complaints such as eczema. Over-indulgence may also cause you to suffer water retention, when you feel swollen and puffy and your ankles swell. Your eyesight will also deteriorate.

Water and fire create bitter nutrients such as green vegetables, coffee and tea. If you feel liverish, nauseated and headachy, these are the substances to take, say the Tibetan doctors. However, if you over-indulge in them you may experience an increase in anxiety and a feeling of over-sensitivity which can make you very insecure. Western dieticians would support these findings. Too much coffee and you can feel very shaky.

A salty taste is created by air and water and is

found in salt, which increases digestive heat, aids the digestive process and gives a good taste to food. Too much, and high blood pressure results as well as wrinkles, hair loss and greying, and a feeling of thirst.

Fire and air make hot tastes as are found in chillies, ginger, radishes, onions, garlic, nutmeg and alcohol. (Tibetans believe that onions encourage sleep onset.) These fiery substances warm your stomach and aid digestion. If you eat too much of them you may lose your libido and if you are a man your sperm count may diminish. Too much of these hot-tasting foods may even interfere with your lung and liver function. If this happens, they say you will feel anxious and frightened with no reason. You may even notice some deterioration in your sight.

Earth and air form astringent-tasting foods such as grapefruit, dandelion leaves, geans, unripe persimmons and turmeric. Though in moderation they clear your complexion, prevent bad breath, encourage bile formation and help headaches, in excess they lead to insomnia, an increase in mucus secretion, increased flatulence, and blocked body channels.

Tibetan medical texts divide food into solid nutrients, such as cooked dishes, meat, vegetables and bread, and liquid foods such as milk, water and alcohol. To remain healthy, to sleep well and have all your bodily functions working normally, they suggest that for each meal you think of your stomach as divided in four. You should fill two parts with solid food, one part with liquid and leave one part for air.

Although the Tibetan diet is very much more limited than in the West, their dietary advice is very similar to Western dietary rules. They also suggest that you should not eat your last meal much later than about 8 p.m. and that you should have a regular time to go to bed, about three hours after the last meal.

This is a medical tradition of 'a place for everything and everything in its place'. It is one that is based on a mixed diet where the different foods are distinguished by their taste which makes it easy for lay people to follow. I find it interesting that the Tibetan medical texts, written so many thousand years ago, knew that sweet foods increase tooth decay, and sour foods such as yoghurt and cheese, if taken in excess, might precipitate eczema. These teachings have only recently become a recognized part of Western medical thought.

If you are sleeping poorly, perhaps you should start by eating a good mixed diet, and go to bed regularly at the same time every night about three hours after your last meal. If you want to follow Tibetan medical thought you should look at your diet, assess whether it is unbalanced and rectify it. You should take some of each of the categories of food every day and if possible all the different tastes of food should be represented in your main meal. Not overeating seems also to be important, as is the balance of liquid to solid food. You may find that as your energy flow and your digestive and body temperature system stabilize your sleep improves. If, after some weeks it has not, then if you want to continue down the Tibetan medical path you should look for a qualified practitioner to prescribe medication for you.

The 'Exegetical Tantra' also speaks about conduct as a healing process. Negativity of mind, action and speech are unbalancing and should be got rid of. You should be impartial, keep your word, refrain from misbehaviour, speak only after thought and generally only do what will benefit society. Work diligently, instructs the Tantra, look after your relations and the elderly and befriend your neighbours. Refrain from envy or the temptation to humiliate and do not work with wicked people even to get a result that you greatly want.

This code of conduct removes stress, guilt and jealousy from your mind and so removes the thoughts which prevent sleep. It is interesting that so many years ago it was also thought to be important. These rules of conduct are worth paying attention to. As for those of you who have not slept, the Tantra dictates that you should miss breakfast and make up half the period of missed sleep. Those of you whose insomnia is dominated by wind should snatch sleep as they can. The old, the depressed, the fearful and the alcoholic should have a siesta in the middle of the day, as should those whose sleep is minimized by long days of hard work in summer. However, normal healthy people should not sleep in the daytime. If you are well and catnap it will increase phlegm and so you may get oedema, colds, contagious fevers and headaches. If you are drowsy all day, the Tantra suggests an emetic or fasting or sexual intercourse to cure it. It goes on to suggest that to cure insomnia you should take warm milk, curd, wine or meat broth before bedtime and allow your head to be massaged with sesame butter and your ears lightly coated with oil. It sounds a good regime to me.

Summary

> While the bee with honied thigh,
> That at her flowery work doth sing,
> And the waters murmuring
> And such concert as they keep,
> Entice the dewy-feathered sleep
>
> *John Milton*

1. Modern Tibetan medical science is built on an ancient tradition whose text is the *Four Tantras*.

2. It is based on keeping your body in balance with itself and all around it.

3. In this way it is similar to and may have had the same origins as Ayurvedic and Chinese medicine.

4. Medicaments are complicated mixtures of herbs and minerals and are given according to the Law of Contraries. Acupuncture and moxibustion are also used in treatment.

5. Conduct and diet are important parts of treatment and maintaining health. In these areas you may follow Tibetan practice.

6. Medication and acupuncture are best left to qualified Tibetan doctors.

Chapter Ten

Special cases

Jet lag

Travel across time upsets your body clock, which gets used to going to sleep, waking and eating at set hours. Short journeys pose little problem. Fly for two hours east and you may lose much of the morning or afternoon or miss four hours' sleep. You can adjust for that by going to bed earlier for some days before. Fly two hours west and you scarcely notice the time change. When it gets to longer journeys there is a greater strain on your body clock. The best way to deal with these journeys is to go to bed as soon as you arrive, set your alarm to allow you two full hours' sleep and then wake, get dressed and continue in the new time zone. How does this work? Take a journey to America. Leave at 9 a.m., arrive at 9 a.m., but the journey is five hours so you feel you have arrived at 2 p.m. body clock time. This is ideal, as your circadian rhythm tends to prepare you for sleep at this time. A two-hour 'crash out' is very natural. You are then full of energy for a slightly longer day than usual but it is always easier to stay up late than wake early.

Going east is never so comfortable. Leave at nine on a five-hour journey and arrive about 7 p.m. though your body clock still tells you it is 2 p.m. Sleep for two hours then get up and enjoy the nightlife in wherever you are. The great thing is to use the circadian dip which occurs every twelve hours to help you regain energy until the next sleep time. When travelling it is wise to take little alcohol or rich fatty foods as these will interfere with your sleep pattern on arrival, and the loss of body fluid due to increased perspiration in the dry atmosphere of the plane tends to make alcohol's side-effects more intrusive. Plenty of water and dilute fruit juice are better travelling companions.

Sleep on that first night in a strange place may be assisted by using any of the methods offered in this book. If things like the classical music cassette, 'Sound Asleep for Adults', a warm glass of barley water, self-massage of the toes and forefoot, or a lavender-scented bath do not help, then a short-acting sleeping pill which does not change your sleep pattern, or, from homeopathy, a Coffea 30c tablet, or a sedative

herbal tea that suits you, or from Chinese
medicine, acupressure, may do the trick.

Shift workers

Any of the above aids to sleep are worth trying
on the night when your shift changes. It is easier
for you to move your shift forward by the clock
and this is worth negotiating with your employ-
ers if they are not already doing it. It is also
better to spend some time in any one shift so
your body clock may adjust: a three-month
change around is probably the minimum time to
prevent a disruptive effect. Many people prefer
to alter their lifestyle for much longer periods
and achieve a happy life with decent sleep,
working at unusual times. Anything less than
three months between shift changes may
become very sleep-disruptive and lead to sleep
deprivation.

I know some people like to do a series of
twelve-hour shifts for part of the week and then
have some days off to be with their family. This
may be socially attractive but it is quite hard to
get your sleep pattern to adjust to it, especially
as you get older.

My advice on moving shift is again to use
your circadian rhythm to facilitate your sleep
change. Say your usual shift runs for eight hours

from 8 a.m. to 4 p.m. When the change comes and you have to start at 4 p.m., get up early, eat a brunch and sleep for four hours before going to work, using your noon 'blip' to help you sleep. Come off shift and take something light, like a plate of porridge and milk, and sleep another four hours to bring you to breakfast. Become a siesta person. Moving from the late shift is easier. Go to sleep a little earlier to give you eight hours before the 8 a.m. start. To start work at twelve midnight, go to bed after lunch at noon and let your siesta time become extended to give you seven hours.

When you change shifts you may need some help from the techniques I have listed in this book. Find what suits you and stick to it. Habit helps sleep onset. In the end I would not discount the idea of a short-acting sleeping pill, which does not disrupt sleep architecture, taken only for a couple of nights every three months. It is better to be well slept and wide awake than have two lost days at each shift change.

Mothers

Mothers of new babies have a difficult time getting enough sleep. Baby wakes at least every four hours needing a feed and changing. Encourage your baby to look forward to being awake by day by playing and talking to him during the daylight hours and keep the night feed and change as short as possible. It is tempting to extend the night feeds and play with baby when he is entirely your own, but he very quickly gets into the habit of expecting this play time and resents it vocally when you want to sleep. Sleep when baby sleeps is good advice and with a first baby this is possible. It is not when you have older children who need to be got up and dressed for school or nursery. Look for at least seven hours' sleep. You will learn to go straight into deep sleep to snatch the benefit.

You may also reset your sleep pattern to have less deep sleep so your baby's cry wakes you easily. This is a habit that is hard to shake off after baby grows and begins to sleep through the night. You change back to your old sleeping pattern by telling yourself that you may now sleep deeply all night because you are not needing to listen for a cry. In the same way it is very helpful to have a time to sleep when you are not responsible for baby. An afternoon's sleep while grannie or a trusted friend looks after your baby is often the way to avoid sleep deprivation.

It is not possible to keep the normal social hours with a new baby in the house. Abandon them to achieve enough sleep to keep you healthy. This period usually only lasts for about six months, after which your baby changes to a more adult pattern of sleeping.

Babies

Normal babies usually sleep if they are healthy, comfortably warm, well fed and have a clean nappy. If yours does not, look for other causes. Some young babies like to be swaddled and tucked in firmly to lie on their backs or sides. Some prefer a little light; some need a dark room. Noise wakens some babies, others will not sleep until they can hear the noise of the family about them. You must work out baby's preferences. It is worth it to get a good sleep. Fit babies, from about three months onward, sometimes howl when they are put to bed. If this is due to their wish to remain in the family circle, you need to offer them guidelines. Countless books talk about putting baby down firmly, letting him howl a little then reinforcing his bed routine and leaving him to cry. This can breed an olympic howler because he gets the wrong message. He thinks you are telling him that if he howls enough you will pick him up and he is able to howl much longer than you are able to stand the noise. 'Sound Asleep for Babies', a cassette of classical music timed at the brain-wave rate of babies going into sleep, put by the bedside and switched on as you say goodnight has been a boon to many mothers and babies. A musical toy that he associates with goodnight is also helpful, as is the radio left on next door. The great thing is not to let him feel that he only has to cry enough to be picked up for more fun.

He doesn't know that he needs good sleep to grow. You must think for him. Sometimes allowing a healthy howler to sleep with a loving grandmother in charge will break the cycle of howling and being picked up. Baby adapts to new rules without loss of face and then forgets to howl once he is back at home. One of my patients brought her mother to stay for a week. She went to the crying baby, changed him without lifting him from the cot, made him comfortable and told him that everyone was asleep. By the end of the week he slept until ten, woke for the change and a drink of milk and then slept for another six to seven hours. His mother told me he was much more cheerful by day and ate better, too.

If a baby who normally sleeps well suddenly does not it is worth finding out why. As he grows past three months baby tends to enter a more adult type of sleep pattern. He may also have difficulty going to sleep and staying asleep if his life pattern is disrupted by, say, a new sibling or a new school or a frightening film on television. Babies and children who snore and sleep on their fronts with their knees pulled up under them and their neck extended usually have enlarged tonsils and adenoids. They are sleeping like this to achieve a better airway and may need their tonsils or adenoids removed. These are just a few special cases which may help. Sleepless babies could fill a book.

Dementia sufferers and their carers

Ask a carer what he or she needs most and 'sleep' is the usual answer. People with Alzheimer's disease and dementia forget the normal daily round and wander day and night. I believe it is not sensible to try to make them conform to our social timetable; better to divide their day in two.

Start with the evening. I see no alternative to offering a patient with dementia a sleeping pill to send them to sleep if they find it difficult to do so. I would use a short-acting modern hypnotic such as zolpidem or zopiclone that does not upset their sleep pattern. They have enough problems in their brains. They do not need to be stunned by heavy hypnotics which depress any cerebration they have. I suggest that carers give this to them at about 11 at night and reinforce its action with acupressure, music, aromatherapy and reflexology. This way carer and patient can sleep for about four or five hours. This does mean that they both get up about five in the morning but then after breakfast and pottering round they may go out and get some exercise together, even do some shopping and come back for early lunch, when if the demented patient will not rest, I again offer a short-acting sleeping pill at a time when the circadian rhythm of both carer and patient tends to produce sleep. Both may get another four hours. At this point if the carer can get a friend or home help to take over, she may get some time to herself when she can shop or go out to visit friends or just feel 'off call'. The carer then comes back to do the evening stint of looking after before bed. If a music cassette such as 'Sound Asleep for Seniors' or homeopathic medication or reflexology massage or herbal teas will allow the dementia sufferer to sleep in the afternoon it is obviously preferable to a sleeping pill, but a restless patient who wanders all day without rest is an impossible task to look after alone. The sleep deprivation that affects carers may make them less sympathetic to their charges and very depressed in themselves. There are times when a regular life and enough sleep bring benefits to both carer and patient and may allow a demented patient to remain at home for longer that he or she would otherwise.

Snoring

> Laugh and the world laughs with you;
> Snore and you sleep alone.
>
> *Anthony Burgess*

Snoring is caused by the sound made by the vibration of tissue along the path of the air as we breathe in. It may be due to nasal problems, such as a deviated septum, polyps, a stuffy nose or enlarged adenoids. It is mainly due to a lax soft palate and a narrow upper throat whose muscle has deteriorated or been replaced by fat deposits following a weight gain. There is also a rare form of laryngeal snoring, where tissue in the larynx vibrates.

Nasal snoring is usually curable either with nose drops that shrink the lining to normal or by surgery to remove polyps or adenoids or straighten a septum.

Nowadays, for the snoring that is caused by a lax soft palate and narrow throat, surgeons also make little laser cuts in the soft palate to allow the healing fibrosis which follows to strengthen it or tell patients to sleep in a mask attached to a positive airways pressure machine that delivers air to the nose at a higher pressure than the ambient and so keeps the soft palate from vibrating and falling back to block the throat. I believe neither of these rather unpleasant courses are necessary if you catch snoring at an early stage and do professional singers' exercises to strengthen your soft palate and widen your upper throat. These exercises are in a singalong cassette called 'Soundless Sleep for Snorers' and are well explained in my book *The Natural Way To Stop Snoring*.

If allowed to continue, snoring may go on to become obstructive sleep apnoea, a serious condition where chronic lack of oxygen through the night begins to affect the brain, the heart and other organs, and then sleeping attached to a constant positive airways pressure machine becomes life-saving.

Grief

Children cry themselves to sleep and so do adults. It is not grief that ruins your sleep after a bereavement but the fear of death, the uncertainty of your financial position, the loss of your social life and friends and the anxiety associated with the beginning of a new stage in your life. Death, divorce, redundancy are all causes of grief and each in its separate way has to be worked through, using the day for thought and the night for sleep. Physical exercise is your friend; your enemy is anxiety. Happy memories will help you; resentment and a desperate wish to have another chance will not.

Think of your personality as an octopus. Every time you lose something or someone dear to you it is like having a bit cut off. Sometimes it is quite a small loss, like the end of a tentacle. It will grow again. Sometimes it is a large part of you that is lost; healing takes a long time and the scar may remain for ever. Healing is helped by sleep and I hope that some part of this book will help allay the anxieties and insecurities of those of you who grieve, so that you may win through to peace of mind.

Stay-at-homes

Nursing home inhabitants who never go outside were found to sleep less well than their age equals who did get out into the sunlight. The stay-at-homes were also found to have lower circulating melatonin levels. The production of melatonin's precursor, melanin, is encouraged by sunlight. Melanin is the colour in our tan. Not only exercise, but exercise in the outdoors where the sun can reach you, seems to help you get a good sleep. This does not mean that you should lie in the sun for long. We know that long exposure to sunlight may encourage skin cancers to occur. It is another case where doing things in moderation is good for you.

From the East came Reiki

Reiki is Japanese for Universal Life Energy and its followers believe that it flows through and around all living things. Reiki Masters seek to activate it to heal your body, mind and spirit. They do this by allowing you to lie relaxed and warm while they lay their hands on either side of your head and face, on your neck and shoulders and where there is pain.

Through their hands runs the Universal Force. They do not control it, it merely flows through them. Thus, in theory, anyone may learn to be a Reike Master. Like Yoga and T.M., you must be taught by a properly qualified teacher and this costs money, although payment may also be in kind.

The Universal Force is not specified. It releases blocked energies, allows your body to cleanse itself from toxins and peps up your personal energy.

Reike Principles counsel: 'Just for today do not anger. Just for today do not worry. Honour your parents, teachers and elders. Earn your living honestly. Show gratitude to every living thing.'

Reike is just one of many theories springing up to offer people peace of mind. It is relaxing to lie with a gentle hand upon you. How seldom do we take the time to do so. Reike workers can even offer Reike to themselves as the Life Force just passes through their hands coming from they know not where and entering the body the hands touch to strengthen its own force to heal itself. If you find comfort and ease from allowing your hands to lie gently on your body then I can see no harm in it. I am always unhappy when not insubstantial payment is demanded because people who may not easily afford it may not receive as much benefit as their outlay warrants. However, if it works for you this is a very gentle non-injurious path to peace of mind and health and sound sleep.

Summary

I really can't be expected to drop everything and start counting sheep at my age. I hate sheep.

Dorothy Parker

1. If you are comfortable in mind and body, well exercised, well fed and healthy you should have no trouble going to sleep.

2. Difficulty in getting to sleep or staying asleep is not a disease in itself. It is the cause of insomnia that should be sought and treated.

3. This book offers many different ways to help you get to sleep. Find some that suit you and build them into a habit to help you get enough sleep to keep you wide awake by day.

4. You have slept as well as you need at night if you don't need to sleep in the day.

5. If you are pregnant or a nursing mother you should ask your doctor before you take any medication of your own for sleep.

6. Children and babies should not be given hypnotic medication unless your doctor has prescribed it or tells you to use it.

Chapter Eleven

An overview

So is sleeplessness a disease?

No it is not. Insomnia is a sign that something has disrupted your normal daily habits. It may be due to a disease, to stress, to a misconception of how much sleep you really need, or an abnormal lifestyle. Depending on which medical approach you accept it may be caused by weakened body resistance, blocked Qi channels or to imbalance of your humoural make up.

Does a poor night's sleep matter?

Yes. It leads to a day when you are more tired than you should be, your reflexes are slower, your judgement suspect, everything you do takes more effort and your mood is sour.

If you only have one bad night you can put up with a rotten day and make up sleep the next night. If the bad nights go on and on you reach a state of short-temperedness, depression and lethargy which affects everything you do. In your personal relationships this may lead to family strife. Your work may suffer and in this car-borne age you may drive recklessly or fall asleep at the wheel.

Chronic sleep deprivation can lead to illness. High blood pressure and heart disease from unrelieved stress; poor body resistance to invading disease and depression are all sequelae to long-term sleep loss.

It is possible to override sleeplessness with stratagems and medication.

If you are being kept awake by the excitement of a coming exam or a job interview, a wedding, a concert or any short-term grief or malaise, these short-term methods to override your insomnia may be enough to keep you going over the bad patch. Afterwards your sleep pattern will return and you will be able to make up the loss over a few nights.

It is not sensible to continue to use the stratagems I have described in previous chapters if your sleep loss persists. You should seek expert advice. It is even less sensible to use hypnotic medication in the long term.

Short-term use of sleeping pills may see you over a bad patch but you should make sure that any you use have no effect on your sleep pattern so that when you stop them your sleep is not disturbed by withdrawal effects.

Hypnotics may find a place in the occasional

use by shift workers at the time of shift change. Jet lag is often more readily treated with herbal remedies or music because you are tired already and just need to 'get over'.

As soon as you realize you have a real problem going to sleep, you should start to deal with it. If you have no idea why it has occurred, see your doctor and allow him to check that you are not unwell. If you are well aware of the cause, and if, for example, it is stress at work or family stress at home, by all means use the short-term stratagems I have described to help you get as much sleep as you can. But realize that you must look into your dilemma and find a solution. It is tempting to allow life to go on in the same rut until catastrophe finally wrecks your unhappy path. By then, chronic sleep loss will leave you unable to make reasonable decisions on how to go on.

Don't let this happen. Look at your own abilities and desires. Make up your mind about what sort of life you want and plan your path through life as far as you can. If you cannot sleep because you are unable to cope with your work or a family relationship, settle down to think out what you can cope with and arrange your life accordingly. This may need serious changes in your lifestyle. You have to make your mind up whether you can tolerate this or whether you want to continue plodding along, tired and miserable.

Remember that if you cannot perform a task or obligation, that is not your fault. You are untrained or unable. Let it become the problem of whoever set you to do the job. Let them worry about it. Clear your mind of the stress that follows overwhelming activities you cannot perform. You will sleep the better for it. There are many ways to slide into sleep comfortably. You don't need to be sleep deprived to use them to make your passage into the restorative activity that we call sleep a pleasant one. A good sleep hygiene routine makes oncoming night a treat to look forward to.

Your body will be motivated to enter sleep if it is physically tired. In addition, exercise helps all your bodily functions, from regularizing your bowel motions to encouraging your circulation. Like all animals you need to give your body activity to keep it healthy. This does not mean you should take sudden, heavy exercise. You should build up to a reasonable amount of exercise that leaves you pleasantly weary at night. Depending on your age and fitness, this may be anything from exercises from a chair or a good walk or swimming to a regular workout in the gym or on the playing field. Manual workers get their exercise at their jobs every day; houseworkers also. Looking after a family keeps you well exercised.

Babies of under six months tire after a half-hour of handling and need to be put to sleep. As they grow their exercise potential increases and one sure way of encouraging your child to sleep well at night is to make sure he or she is physically tired, but not overtired, by bedtime.

Many of you have sedentary jobs and only exercise at the weekends. This sort of exceptional exercise after a week of lethargy is not especially good for your bodies and a more regular exercising pattern should be beneficial. Walking to work and back is one way to do this, or going for a walk when you first return home. If you are in doubt about your ability to take exercise, seek professional advice from your doctor.

Never exercise just before bedtime as the adrenalin rush you experience with exercise tends to counter sleep onset. However, if your body is tired it will want to enter sleep.

Try some of the techniques I have described, from aromatherapy to diet, to make bed a place to look forward to, confident that you have a comfortable quiet bedroom, a quiet mind and are tired enough to sleep. You will then be able to give of your best the next day.